EMOTIONALLY FOCUSED
THERAPY FOR TRAUMA

Also from Susan M. Johnson
and published by The Guilford Press

Attachment Processes in Couple and Family Therapy
Edited by Susan M. Johnson and Valerie E. Whiffen

*Attachment Theory in Practice: Emotionally Focused Therapy (EFT)
with Individuals, Couples, and Families*
Susan M. Johnson

*Emotionally Focused Couple Therapy with Trauma Survivors:
Strengthening Attachment Bonds*
Susan M. Johnson

Emotionally Focused Therapy for Couples
Leslie S. Greenberg and Susan M. Johnson

Emotionally Focused Therapy for Trauma

Susan M. Johnson
T. Leanne Campbell

THE GUILFORD PRESS
New York   London

Printed in the United States of America

This book is printed on acid-free paper.

For product and safety concerns within the EU, please contact
GPSR@taylorandfrancis.com, Taylor & Francis Verlag GmbH,
Kaufingerstraße 24, 80331 München, Germany.

Last digit is print number: 9 8 7 6 5 4 3 2

This publication is intended to provide helpful and informative material. It is not
intended to diagnose, treat, cure, or prevent any health problem or condition, nor
is it intended to replace the advice of a health professional. No action should be
taken based solely on the contents of this book. Always consult your physician
or qualified health care professional on any matters regarding your health and
before adopting any suggestions in this book or drawing inferences from it.

The authors and publisher specifically disclaim all responsibility for any
liability, loss, or risk, personal or otherwise, which is incurred as a consequence,
directly or indirectly, from the use or application of any contents of this book.

Any and all product names referenced within this book are the trademarks
of their respective owners. Always read all information provided by the
manufacturers' product labels before using their products. The authors and
publisher are not responsible for claims made by manufacturers.

Library of Congress Cataloging-in-Publication Data is available from the
publisher.

ISBN 978-1-4625-5929-9 (hardcover)

To our families,

John, Tim (Matteo), Sarah
(Kelly and granddaughter Amelie), and Emma.
—Sue

Darren and Emma.
—Leanne

And to our clients and colleagues
who continually teach and inspire us.

About the Authors

Susan M. Johnson, EdD, until her death in 2024, was Professor Emeritus of Clinical Psychology at the University of Ottawa, Ontario, Canada; Distinguished Research Professor in the Marriage and Family Therapy Program at Alliant International University in San Diego; and Director of the International Centre for Excellence in Emotionally Focused Therapy (ICEEFT). "Dr. Sue" was the pioneering innovator of emotionally focused therapy (EFT). She published widely, including acclaimed books for professionals, bestselling books for general readers, and numerous articles, book chapters, and teaching videos. Her seminal contributions to couple therapy have been recognized with the Family Psychologist of the Year Award from Division 43 of the American Psychological Association and the Outstanding Contribution to Marriage and Family Therapy Award from the American Association for Marriage and Family Therapy. She was most proud of receiving the Order of Canada, one of the country's highest civilian honors.

T. Leanne Campbell, PhD, is cofounder and managing partner of Campbell & Fairweather Psychology Group, a multisite clinical practice in British Columbia, Canada. She is an executive board member of the ICEEFT and an ICEEFT Certified Trainer, also serving as site coordinator for a large-scale study examining the efficacy of emotionally focused individual therapy (EFIT). Dr. Campbell is an international speaker, writer, trainer, and codeveloper of EFT-related educational programs and materials. She has coauthored several peer-reviewed articles and books on EFT, most notably the first seminal text on EFIT, *A Primer for Emotionally Focused Individual Therapy* (with Susan M. Johnson), now translated into multiple languages.

Preface

This book is the culmination of our work together over the past years, of what we have learned from working with couples, from over three decades of emotionally focused couple therapy research, from our pioneering research on emotionally focused individual therapy, and from our many colleagues and leaders in the trauma and psychotherapy fields who have similarly devoted themselves to these important topics over the course of their careers. It also represents our work with thousands of individuals, couples, and families over the past decades.

The people you will meet in this book represent clients and composites of many people we have worked with and, in some cases, summaries of various client stories that have been shared with us. In such latter cases, we have used gender-neutral pronouns. In the case of transcripts, the pronouns we have used are those used by the clients. As well, while protecting the confidentiality of our clients, we have mainly preserved the transcripts as they occurred in session, edited only for the purposes of brevity, clarity, and client confidentiality.

We are grateful to all our clients for the stories they have shared, and the hope and inspiration they have provided.

We also recognize that elements of these clients' experiences might, in some ways, match your own. We invite you to read with attention to your own self-care and with compassion for your own experiences.

As a final note, while this book was well underway prior to losing Sue to cancer in 2024, she did not live to see it published. Sue was confident in its completion, however, and hopeful of the impact it would have on the lives of many. Often referencing the words of Mary Oliver, "Tell me, what is it you plan to do with your one wild and precious life?," her work is a testament to the answer: a lot! As she had planned to do, Sue lived fully until she died. This book is among her last professional contributions. We honor her legacy and are grateful for the many ways Sue has and will continue to impact the lives of so many around the globe!

Acknowledgments

Once again, we are grateful for the generosity of so many clients who have described their experiences of increased hope and healing so we could share them in this book. Of course, we have disguised these contributions to protect the clients' confidentiality. We wish to thank the many others who have supported our work more generally, and specifically with this book: therapists from around the globe who sparked dialogue and growth with thoughtful and on-target questions and commentary, and participants in our trainings who have done the same; the various hosts who have brought these audiences to us; the creative and dedicated global community of ICEEFT (International Centre for Excellence in Emotionally Focused Therapy) trainers and supervisors whose writing, research, training, and mentorship have contributed globally to the growth of the EFT (emotionally focused therapy) model and its accessibility and applicability; and a growing number of inspiring ICEEFT community leaders who uphold the vision and mission of growth in connection, and who have invited us into their communities to train and grow alongside them.

A special thank you to Jackie Evans, our trusted editor and organizer extraordinaire, for your contributions to this book, and many others—we are grateful for your dedication to precision, consistency, and clarity! Thank you as well to Emma Kiedyk, an EFT therapist-in-training who read every chapter with an eye not only on the details, but also on the accessibility of the book for new and seasoned clinicians alike. And, of course, we are grateful to the staff at The Guilford Press: Jim Nageotte, who has worked on other EFT-related publications over the years, his colleague Jane Keislar, and the entire Guilford team.

And thank YOU for joining us! We hope that you will be as inspired as we have been! If you are new to EFT, we hope you will continue to grow alongside us. If EFT is familiar, welcome back! We hope this book will add to your repertoire of skills and understanding of trauma, and that the magic and power, the art and science, of psychotherapy continues to captivate and move you, and your clients!

Contents

Chapter 1   Transforming Trauma Together   1
with Emotionally Focused Therapy

Chapter 2   Attachment Science as the Path to Healing   15

Chapter 3   The Five EFT Macro Interventions   33

Chapter 4   Key EFT Assumptions and Micro Interventions   52

Chapter 5   Assessment as a Guide through the Three Stages   70
of EFIT Intervention

Chapter 6   Finding Focus and Maintaining Momentum in Stage 1   106

Chapter 7   Harnessing Connection to Dissolve Shame in Stage 2   135

Chapter 8   Consolidation in Stage 3   174

Chapter 9   Addressing Other Types of Trauma with EFIT   197

Contents

Appendix   Moving through the Three Stages of EFIT   219

           References   237

           Index   243

1

Transforming Trauma Together with Emotionally Focused Therapy

All of us, at some time in our lives, need the help of others to deal well with our vulnerabilitiy. Life is trouble, the Buddhist teacher Jack Kornfield reminds us. It is also inevitably an encounter with terrifying uncertainty and loss. For the lucky few, these moments are fleeting and melt into a mosaic of comfort and confidence—our frailty becomes manageable. But for many, they morph into a dragon that stalks our dreams and hijacks our waking hours.

People often seek out the help of a therapist in these times, when their emotional pain can no longer be endured or when their way of coping with this pain becomes a problem in itself. In session, Ellen tells her therapist that she is so numb that she is hardly alive, and her only emotion is "irritation." Sunita says she is paralysed and caught in a state of constant planning and rumination interspersed with panic attacks, especially when she thinks of interacting with people. Dealing with human dilemmas around vulnerability is a therapist's stock in trade. Clients vary wildly, of course, in their resources, level of resilience, and the nature of triggering events in their lives. The most natural healing arena for any trauma is in the arms of someone you love, but many of us are still searching for that someone or do not know how to let supportive others in. There are limited ways to cope with human frailty. If not seeking to be seen and held, then we pray, meditate, exercise, recite poetry that adds meaning to a moment, write in a journal, or seek a wiser other: priest, seer, celebrity, or therapist.

In general, mental health professionals' increasing focus on traumatic events and their echoes as core mechanisms of mental and emotional problems seems to represent a shift from a key focus on inner personality

1

factors to a greater acknowledgment of the impact of external events. This is especially true with relational dramas where we are starved of the safe emotional connection with another that we all long for. A popular book, *What Happened to You?: Conversations on Trauma, Resilience, and Healing,* suggests that the key question for those struggling in the wake of traumatic experiences may not be "Who are you inside?" but "What happened to you?" (Perry & Winfrey, 2021). Attachment science suggests that many so-called dysfunctional responses are, in fact, not personality flaws but distortions of natural positive coping responses to impossible situations, where a truly functional solution to annihilating vulnerability was not to be found. These dysfunctional responses become habitual and automatic, and, literally, create a trauma trap, that is a pattern of triggers and coping responses that perpetuate emotional problems and prevent growth.

Henny described her life as a "whirlwind" and indeed, she spoke very fast, moving from story to story and from childhood to recent events in an intellectualized, haphazard way that was very difficult to make sense of. In initial sessions, she and her therapist struggled to piece together key events and timelines for childhood experiences and for more recent events, including a breakup. Most of the first 10 sessions were spent in empathic reflection mode, clarifying key moments in Henny's emotional life and how she dealt with these moments, and also the patterns in how she engaged with others in her life.

For most of us the word *trauma* conjures up an image of an overwhelming, life-changing event or a series of events that induce terror and helplessness—an emotional reaction that is burned into the nervous system of the victim and cannot help but have a lasting impact. The word itself comes from a Greek word meaning "to wound." This encounter with intense helplessness often shifts the existential axis of our world, imprinting us in a way that irrevocably shapes and changes how we see life itself and our sense of who we are, especially our sense of control, worth, and competence. *Traumatic experience is not just painful, it changes how we engage with ourselves and our world.* Some of us can integrate and grow from this experience, but some of us become stuck in recurring darkness. For these latter folks, what felt predictable becomes random, what felt safe becomes imbued with threat, what was manageable becomes a tsunami, what was potentially tolerable becomes a frantic search for escape.

WHERE ARE WE NOW IN OUR PERSPECTIVE ON TRAUMA?

Our view of trauma and the chaos it brings in its wake has changed. As Bessel van der Kolk notes in his splendid book on trauma, *The Body*

Keeps the Score (2015), "We are on the verge of becoming a trauma-conscious society." It is hard to remember that only a couple of decades ago, psychology textbooks would note that trauma was something that happened to only 1% of people, and the formal diagnosis of posttraumatic stress disorder (PTSD) was relatively rare. We now know that, in fact, up to 70% of us will experience at least one traumatic event in our lives, and many of us may go on to develop some or the full gamut of stress disorder symptoms and to be formally diagnosed with PTSD. In the course of a lifetime, 1 in 13 people will likely develop mild to severe PTSD, often with accompanying symptoms such as chronic depression. For some kinds of trauma, such as rape, these numbers are much higher—almost half of these clients go on to display full-blown PTSD. We have also become increasingly more aware of the devastating effects of early trauma, often called *developmental trauma*. Such wounds are most often inflicted by those who a child counts on for security and nurturing. The experience of suffering such wounds often results in what most clinicians call *complex PTSD*. Just a superficial glance at these effects, such as ongoing difficulties in trusting others and a deep fear that one is somehow contaminated, defective, and at fault, gives us a sense of how such trauma can undermine the very basis of any competent or acceptable sense of self.

We seem to have come full circle from minimizing the extent of traumatic experience to recognizing just how common traumatic experience is. We are also recognizing how many people encounter a cascade of traumatic experiences, beginning in childhood (Felitti et al., 1998), that sap physical and emotional vitality and render us more susceptible to ongoing trauma in adulthood.

The general public awareness of trauma and its impacts has changed significantly in the last decade, from a focus on pathology (the reification of the stance, "If you can't get over it then there is something wrong with you"), to a more *existential focus*. Specifically, experiences such as random violence, rape, childhood abuse of all kinds, the wounds of war and those of first responders, as well as traumas due to repeated discrimination, rejection, and abandonment, are now widely recognized as toxic, ubiquitous, and potentially self-perpetuating in nature.

As clinicians, we see how traumatic experience assaults our fragile sense of order and control, and pushes us headlong into a dance with the four existential demons that we all face (Yalom, 1980): the terror of death, along with a sense of our finiteness and the inevitability of loss; the need to shape meaning—a sense that one's life matters—into a short and often seemingly random life path; the dilemma of making choices when uncertainty and threat are everywhere; and the fear of isolation and not mattering to others. Amy tells her therapist, "I can't sleep, even now, 20 years later. I need all the lights on and noise. Those nights locked in my room, alone in the dark as a child, were like death. What is the point? I can't escape this . . . this . . . horror. It comes for me. So, I don't eat and that helps me numb out. I want to connect with people but can't do it in the end. I hide in fear. I am always alone, and the more alone I feel, the more I hide."

We are also now recognizing the multidimensional nature of the impacts of trauma, both acute and chronic developmental trauma, and how it underlies and primes many other problems, such as addiction, chronic depression, and anxiety disorders. Some 70% of those diagnosed with PTSD also meet the criteria for serious depression. In short, our understanding of the phenomena of trauma and the injuries it inflicts has mushroomed in the last decade (Winfrey & Perry, 2021). Research has shown us that trauma creates huge difficulties in being able to deal with, grasp, and accept one's emotions. Pierre Janet, one of the great pioneers in the trauma field, defined PTSD as a disorder of "vehement emotions." In general, it is accepted that "stress exposure is an inherently emotional experience and an individual's ability to regulate their emotional response plays an essential role in their susceptibility or resilience to adversity" (Freidman et al., 2021). Traumatic experience also narrows attention, negatively impacting effective information processing and the maintenance of a coherent perspective. Attention is constrained by a constant vigilance for threat, as is the creation of a confident and competent sense of self. All of which, of course, get in the way of being able to explore, learn, grow, and adapt to new situations—that is, to leave the trauma in the past and live actively in the present. In our session, Ellen acknowledges, "I don't really take in much. I am on autopilot. I just check my body for signs of panic and watch for danger around every corner, in every face."

In the last two decades we have also learned much about the nature of resilience and the factors that can protect us from the pernicious effects of traumatic experience. We can note general personality factors such as optimism and openness to experience (Bonanno et al., 2011), as well as a sense of meaning and purpose in life, and a commitment to religion and spirituality. The two factors that really stand out are, again, the ability to regulate emotion and the presence and quality of supportive social networks—especially the felt presence of an attachment figure with whom a person has a sense of secure connection. It is the factor of having the support of a secure attachment figure that predicted resilience in the survivors of the 9/11 tragedy in New York (Fraley et al., 2006). In fact, secure bonds with others appear to predict better mental health and a lower susceptibility to every psychological disorder!

The most pressing question in the field now appears to be, "How do we begin to effectively heal the aftereffects of traumatic experience?"

We know that some factors, like physical activity and exercise, can help modulate stress, down regulating the nervous system, increasing compounds that affect mood like dopamine, and decreasing stress hormones, like cortisol (Averill et al., 2021). But the question still remains, "What is necessary and sufficient to get to the heart of the matter and significantly transform or bring closure to the echoes of trauma?" What must happen for Henny, sexually and physically abused by her father in her youth with no recourse or island of safety, to be able to access the core of her trauma, tolerate it, and move into and through it in a way that changes her relationship to her dreadful history, and also the relationship to herself and to others?

HOW DO WE BEST TREAT TRAUMATIC STRESS?

Even with the increased attention the field has given to trauma and its impact on human beings, the key question of how to help people heal from trauma is still hanging in the balance. There are a myriad of different interventions to address various elements that are viewed as maintaining posttraumatic symptoms and blocking movement into growth and resilience. However, the core, necessary, and sufficient factors that determine recovery, that offer the promise of a sense of competence in managing threat and closure to past wounds, are still vague in much of the psychological and psychotherapy literature. People tell therapists that they spend their lives doing yoga and mindfulness practices, acupuncture and exercise programs, which all help to reduce stress and awaken their bodies, but they still cannot break the tenacious grip that trauma has over their emotional realities, their minds, and their relationships.

It is useful to consider the difference between different levels of change. The Austrian biologist, Ludwig von Bertalanffy, who wrote in the 1960s about how living systems worked, suggested that there are two levels of change. First-level change modifies various individual elements or parts of a system, such as building specific muscles in someone's legs or finding a more positive thought to replace a negative one, perhaps reducing the stress hormone, cortisol. Second-level change, on the other hand, addresses the organization of the system as a whole and involves a reorganization of self-maintaining patterns and ingrained habits into a new whole. This concept really helped me (Sue), as a crazy young graduate student, to sort through all kinds of changes in client symptoms that different models of therapy measured, and to keep asking the question "What are the core elements that *have* to change to really make a difference to this client?" This sparked an even bigger question: "What kind of change is the therapist really supposed to go for—a reduction in symptoms, less negative thoughts, or maybe even a more fully flexible, growing and alive client?" The last answer seemed pretentious, at the time, but after 35 years of practice and research in emotionally focused therapy (EFT), for couples (EFCT), and for individuals (EFIT), perhaps we can, after all, now embrace it.

How do we grasp the core organizing elements that we need to focus on to transform the echoes of trauma? Do we look at labels from the American Psychiatric Association's DSM-5-TR or from the World Health Organization's ICD-11? These labels tend to be abstract and confusingly overlap. If, instead, we stay close to our traumatized clients, how do they describe their experience? Again and again, we hear:

• *Despair about ongoing, overwhelming emotional pain that cannot be managed.* Clients repeatedly tell us, "I am in chaos, always overwhelmed; all these negative feelings hijack me. I cannot tolerate this or find a way to make sense of it. I spend my whole life trying to shut down my inner demons." Fear predominates here to the point where this emotion is scary in itself. Sarah says, "I cannot count on me at all. If I get triggered, I lose it."

• *Crushing emotional isolation and loneliness.* Statements like the following abound: "I am so alone." "I am unseen, invisible." "Nobody cared or cares about me." "I am not important." "I do not matter to anyone." Sadness and longing are the dominant emotions here, often hidden beneath anger or apparent indifference. Negative cognitive models of others also make opening up impossibly risky. Tara says, "My husband loves me. He is great. But when I am upset, I just barricade myself in my room and shut him out."

• *The negative self-sustaining impact of trying to cope with the above experiences on meaning making and sense of purpose.* Saul states, "I am empty. I am so frozen most of the time. I am shut down or just watching for danger cues to the point that I am hardly alive. I live in a fog, numbed out or preparing for the next freak out. There is no point to my life."

• *The lack of connection with a coherent acceptable sense of self.* Amy tells us, "I am crazy. Just so defective and damaged. How did I let these things happen to me? I hide out because I don't want anyone to see me. I don't want you to see me. You will think I am disgusting." Shame and self-denigration are a constant here.

Each of these negative emotional states builds on and feeds the others and induces helplessness and lack of agency. The result is a recurring cascade—a treadmill of threat cues, emotional chaos triggering dysfunctional coping, and alienation from self and others. The impact of secrecy and stigma can also be added to the emerging picture here. It is worth stating that twice as many women get diagnosed with PTSD as men and the best predictor of PTSD is sexual abuse before the age of 18. As Ellen reminds her therapist, "I had to suffer in silence, to save the family. No one wanted to know about my pain, and when it was revealed, it was called a mistake. It was dismissed as unimportant, or I was questioned as to why I had 'let it happen.' Never mind that it started when I was 8 years old."

The key organizing factor in the ongoing set of processes that constitute PTSD, the patterned processes that must be modified in effective therapy, appears to be, first and foremost, the nature and dysregulation of compelling negative emotions. Modifying these processes first requires the creation of a sense of safe connection with a therapist—the supportive other who creates safety as the dragon roars into the client's view.

The second organizing factor that arises from these client's descriptions of their experience is a disturbance in identity, a negative (or incoherent) internal model of self. The self is seen as alien, not belonging with others, and unacceptable to others. Trauma survivors do not feel in charge of their bodies, cognitions, emotions, or interactions with others. This negative view of self often renders them incapable of making the open, safe connections with others that are key to the healing process.

So how does a therapist, in a series of therapy sessions, bring about these core second-order changes? All well-known and tested treatments seem to set up encounters or include some kind of exposure to traumatic memories. The purpose is most often stated in terms of helping clients discover that the trauma is in the past and now tolerable and assisting them in re-evaluating negative thoughts associated with the trauma. Descriptions of interventions such as prolonged exposure (PE), cognitive processing therapy (CPT), cognitive-behavioral therapy (CBT), and eye movement desensitization and reprocessing therapy (EMDR) can be found in the third edition of *Handbook of PTSD: Science and Practice* (Friedman et al., 2021). Some, such as CPT and CBT, focus, more than others, on challenging distorted thoughts arising from trauma. EMDR focuses on reprocessing toxic stored memories, theoretically, by using eye movements guided by the therapist's hands to help integrate these memories. With all assessments of improvement, there are issues due to factors such as whether treatment protocols are faithfully implemented and varying dropout rates. In clinical care, dropout rates seem to range from 38 to 68% (Kehle, 2016). Interestingly, the problem of emotion regulation seems to be mainly targeted by attempts to habituate clients to fear and encouraging new thoughts, termed *cognitive reappraisal*. All of these approaches recognize that in those with PTSD, fear does not seem to extinguish with time, but in fact, generalizes, so that even objectively safe situations are seen as threatening, leaving people beset with increased vigilance for and sensitivity to threat.

Experts agree that PTSD is essentially an emotional disorder, and we suggest that, like depression and anxiety, PTSD fits with the specific outline of such a disorder as presented by behaviorist David Barlow and by EFIT. To experiential therapists such as ourselves, treatment based on those other approaches generally seems to skirt around emotion, rather than address it directly, and use its power to shape positive change. As Carl Rogers put it, all treatments, in some sense, try to "discover the order in experience." Most seem to do this from a cognitive distance, rather than accurately attuning to and diving into the client's lived experience and following what we refer to as "the hot trail of emotion" to get to the heart of the matter.

As we will present in this book, our clients show us that the core of change with traumatized people is captured by the tried-and-true phrase, a *corrective emotional experience*. This was coined by psychoanalyst Franz Alexander in the 1940s to identify the essential curative element in psychotherapy. Such an experience, an *emotional epiphany* if you will, does not simply expose or habituate clients to the key aspects of their trauma, or offer them insight or a coping technique. It restructures the experience—adding to it and configuring it in a way that leads to growth, rather than paralysis. This must be done in a way that sings to the emotional processing center of the brain and sends a message that the client's nervous system is biologically prepared to hear, will code as supremely relevant, and will hold onto. Such an experience restores emotional balance, elicits core emotions, and shapes a new *identity drama*— a new narrative of the self, a new way of seeing and connecting with the self. Saul, a war vet, shares, "I can name it and hold it in my hand now, all that self-disgust. I see that it is deep sadness and longing, really. I can even feel compassion for the solider who limped from the battlefield as a failure—a traitor. That is new—that is heresy for the old Saul, but does it ever feel good. I can believe in me again."

More than three decades of practice and research has taught EFT therapists how to target and shape these emotional epiphanies with consistency and precision. In our research, these events—captured on video, coded, and verified—predict shifts in both distressing symptoms, and in personality growth and resilience (Burgess-Moser, 2012; Dalgleish et al., 2015; Burgess-Moser et al., 2017; Spengler et al., 2024). They create a positive cascade of openness to experience, to self and others, and the ability to engage with and respond to new situations.

HOW DID WE DISCOVER
THESE POTENT CORRECTIVE EXPERIENCES?

Earlier in my career, I (Sue) became obsessed with helping couples find a way through conflict to connection. This idea held my interest, perhaps because no one seemed to know how to do it, but also because it was like solving my parent's fights—the nightmare of my childhood and the tragedy of my father's life. However, I also saw individual clients, such as war vets suffering from flashbacks and depression. At a certain point, women diagnosed with a myriad of different disorders, began turning up in my office with horrific stories of childhood sexual abuse. Female partners in distressed couples also disclosed issues with intimacy and trust, arising from sexual abuse by men in their families of origin. My reaction was to be appalled, angry, and overwhelmed. What could I do to help these clients? The topic of early sexual abuse by fathers, uncles, and brothers, had never even been mentioned in my graduate program! I remember a severely anorexic client came to me who had been through the best treatment program in my city. She told me her history and, in a voice filled with pain, noted that she had shared her abuse in the program but that it had not been commented on. I was thunderstruck, but then I thought, "We don't know how to respond, how to help these folks, so we just screen this out—much as Freud did all those years ago in Vienna."

At the beginning of my recognition of this clinical need, the client who taught me the most was Paula. She came because every morning she had to walk across a bridge over a canal to get to work. In the middle of the bridge, she would be overcome with severe panic and become so dizzy that she had to literally crawl across on her hands and knees to get to the other side. She was also experiencing "rage storms" at her teenage daughter, and she admitted to regularly taking four times the maximum recommended amount of an antianxiety medication, given to her by her GP for her "nerves." I could not understand how she was even walking. As I focused on what happened on the bridge, she gradually revealed that the cars coming toward her felt like missiles about to smash into her and that the space under the bridge seemed to be hundreds of feet deep. She suggested that she was simply "crazy" and losing her mind. Already using the set of interventions that became the EFT model, I did all I could to help her feel safe with me and noted her strengths: She faced the bridge going to work every day and was competent in her job. She kept silent about these panic episodes and the strange images that kept her awake at night in an effort to "protect" her "kind" husband of 25 years and her teenage daughter from their impact. We noted places where she felt safe and relaxed—being in a hot bath with the door locked and candlelight was her best refuge. She had finally confided in her sister, who told her to come to me, and she had found the courage to come! Her problems had worsened as her daughter grew up and reminded Paula of how she looked in early adolescence.

I began to feel my way into Paula's world—her emotional ups and downs, her descriptions of who she was, and her stories of her key relationships. When she talked about her upbringing, she seemed distant and vague, but when she mentioned her mother, she always brushed her hand across her body in what seemed like dismissal. Her family were very religious and her older sister was always destined for the convent, which she entered and stayed in for more than a decade. She noted that her sister had a deadbolt on the inside of her bedroom door, but there was no deadbolt on Paula's door. Her parents split up when she was about 13 and she had then lived alone with her mother with a series of lodgers. Her father had died when she was about 15. A little lost as to how best to help, I did what I was learning to do with distressed couples: I followed and stayed with the most powerful thing in the room, the emotion. I intentionally slowed and lowered my voice to offer a sense of comfort and acceptance, holding and regulating the emotion as I followed, reflected, and explored it with Paula. I already knew how to identify the key elements in the flow of emotional experience and merge them into a coherent whole, reaching for the pain under the reactive surface emotion, which was often anger or simply a numb emptiness.

I began to focus on her vague distant style as she talked about her childhood and the fragmented images that assailed her at night. She remembered, in vivid detail, the wallpaper in her childhood bedroom. This image brought waves of terror, and she began to piece together a sense of how she "went into" the pattern of the wallpaper to escape the "fire" in her body and the feeling of being pinned down. Specific memories now emerged in our sessions, such as being roughly picked up and washed in the kitchen sink by her mother, who kept shouting at her father, "How could you?" A clear picture of her childhood abuse by her father (and later by the various lodgers mentioned above) then emerged, together with her mother's inaction and inability to comfort or protect her. Paula taught me many things, but mostly she taught me to follow my mentors, Rogers and Bowlby, and to accept her truth as it unfurled. I thought we would spend much of our time dealing with fear in many forms. In fact, we spent most of our time grieving for her childhood pain, longings, and isolation. Together we also learned how to build islands of comfort as places of refuge. Paula's nightly bath became an elaborate ritual of calm and connection with herself. As I accepted and went into her pain with her, she began to feel less ashamed and "contaminated," and became more emotionally balanced. She reduced her anxiety medication and found she could walk across the bridge to her workplace, looking ahead and reassuring herself all the way. She brought her husband into two sessions and told him what she had been struggling with all these years. She admitted that she had never actually been present in their lovemaking. She had always been in the wallpaper. They wept together and she was able to tell him how to hold and comfort her. Paula began to experience herself as competent, able to order and deal with her inner chaos and pain.

As we moved into the second stage of therapy, the restructuring of the patterns of emotional experience and the deepening of engagement in core emotions, it seemed natural to ask Paula to do a form of the "softening" conversations that we were finding so transforming in our couple therapy sessions (Johnson 2008, 2020). In these conversations, core vulnerabilities are owned and enacted in a relational context. In this case, the enactment was not with a partner as in couple therapy, but with the key attachment figures that were alive in Paula's mind and heart. We all have constant conversations with such figures, and it is in this context that we constantly decide who we are and how worthy we are. I had assumed that this new emotional experience, the new emotional music when turned into a dance with another, would involve Paula's father, but very often therapy does not move in the direction of confronting the abuser or those involved in the actual traumatic experience. As Paula moved into and through her grief at being abandoned and used, the terror and threat cues that still hijacked her, and her sense of shame, it was her mother that became alive in the room. Paula still looked for birthday cards from her now aged mother, but they never came. As Paula played out her now clear and coherent response to her mother's abandonment and denial of her pain, she became more assertive and confident. She ended up traveling across the country and confronting her mother in person, not expecting a healing response, but as a way of standing with the small, vulnerable part of herself that she had contacted and held and learned to value in our sessions.

By the end of therapy, Paula no longer had panic attacks or nightmares, could relate to her adolescent daughter on a different level, and confide in and receive comfort from her husband. I became more and more caught up in my quest to develop a truly effective couple therapy, to come up with a definitive solution to relationship distress and lack of secure attachment in couples. I learned so much and continued to practice with individual survivors until the pressure to explicate, write about, and research EFIT—how we helped people move out of the trap of trauma, anxiety, and depression—could no longer be resisted.

WHAT ARE THE CORE ELEMENTS IN TRAUMA RECOVERY?

What stands out from our observation of countless video sessions, clinical practice, and client stories is that recovery involves:

- A more open and deeper level of engagement in one's emotional experience, including the ability to access, tolerate, and ORDER this experience, increasing emotional balance and coherent information processing.
- Several increasingly significant, absorbing corrective emotional epiphanies that address the helplessness and loss provoked by the client's trauma. Inevitably, these emotional epiphanies address the core emotions of sadness and longing, shame and fear.
- A restructuring of the client's model of self into a new sense of competence, worth, and agency. This restructuring may be formulated as the creation of a secure sense of connection with a now accepted and acceptable self.
- The creation of more engaged and supportive relationships with others, including the ability to reach for others when vulnerable, to trust them, and be able to take in their reassurance.

However, to truly understand vulnerability with no solution and how to deal with it, we must first understand the nature of human fear. Attachment science offers us this understanding. It gives us a profound way of grasping human suffering that allows us to shape the pathway to further development and growth. The intervention technology acquired in the practice and study of EFT also gives us the specific tools to effectively work into and through that suffering, whether it is our own or that of others. This book will elaborate on both attachment science and the techniques of EFT.

WE HOPE TO INSPIRE YOU
AS OUR CLIENTS HAVE INSPIRED US

We seem to mostly grasp enormous, multifaceted realities mainly through stories, images, and metaphors, so you will encounter many here.

A metaphor, taken from Celtic mythology, to capture the experience of trauma was previously used to open a book on EFT with traumatized couples (Johnson, 2002). In the Celtic stories, life is portrayed in dark terms indeed. This metaphor is about standing in a dark, narrow passageway with your back against a wall, facing a dragon. There is no escape. For the Celts, a warrior people, the only question is how well you fight.

There is also a famous Buddhist story (Pema Chodron, 2002) that describes life in terms of a woman running from tigers. She runs but the tigers get closer. She comes to the edge of a cliff. She sees a vine, and climbing over the cliff, holds onto it. Then she sees that there are tigers below her as well. She then notices that a mouse is gnawing away at the vine she is holding onto. As she turns her head, she sees a beautiful clump of ripe strawberries growing just beside her. She looks up and down, and at the mouse. Then she reaches for a strawberry, pops it in her mouth, and enjoys it thoroughly.

Both stories paint dark threats and deep vulnerability as unavoidable. In existential terms, if we see it clearly, life is filled with terrors. We all face the same monsters. Some of us become consumed by these monsters. Nevertheless, many of us manage to deal well with these threats and various moments of fragility. We find ourselves able to access our strength and fight against overwhelming odds. We find ourselves still able to feel the sun on our face and to reach for joy. Our clients have taught us—and can teach all of us—how to find the strength to face the dragon of trauma well and how to reach past it for joy and aliveness.

In the first half of this book, you will learn how to understand traumatic experience through the lens of attachment theory and science—a science of how we get stuck in dark places and how we let in the light and grow. Attachment links our biology to the ways we see the world and dance with others, and that is a fascinating intellectual leap. There is a structure to our nervous system, to our emotions, and to the ways we deal with helplessness. Once we grasp the structure, it is easier to change it. You will also learn about how therapists using EFT tune into their clients and use a certain vision, a way of seeing, to kick-start change.

In Chapters 3 and 4, we offer a summary of what EFT therapists actually do in a session and how these interventions impact those who come for help. We hope these chapters will particularly appeal to health professionals, but we think it's relevant for all of us to know the techniques and moves that have been shown to help folks face dragons and emerge, not just intact, but whole. We share our clients' stories and offer you snapshots of therapy sessions to help you connect with these brave people and so learn from them as we have.

In the second half of the book, we will introduce you to clients facing different kinds of trauma and show you how therapist and client come together to transform the echoes of trauma on the level of emotional patterns, connection with others, and how the self is defined. We know you will enjoy meeting them and that you will see yourself and your life in their struggles.

Finally, we will share with you what we see as the promise of the vision laid out in this book. This is the promise that resilience is our birthright and that there is a way home for any of us, once we find the path through the darkness and the mist.

We hope to inspire you, offer you hope, and maybe even capture your heart with our stories. We believe passionately in psychotherapy, which is a refined and deliberate elaboration on the natural healing power of safe relationships and the healthy ways our species has of facing overwhelming challenge and lack of control, and of reaching for aliveness in the face of impossible odds.

It helps us all to know how survivors grow and thrive, and how to aid them on their way. It helps all of us to know how to hold and grow the most vulnerable and wounded part of ourselves.

2

Attachment Science
as the Path to Healing

Sometime in the 1930s, a rather uptight, young aristocratic Englishman, who would go on to be a prominent psychiatrist and leader in the field of psychotherapy, must have walked through the streets of London, seeing the delinquents of that city, usually regarded simply as criminals requiring punishment, and noting the desperation and pain hidden behind their aggressive behavior. This was John Bowlby. He saw past their protective façades to their inner vulnerability. He began to work with delinquent children and became fascinated by how experiences of loss and separation from their parents was such a common factor in their lives. He began to fight with the analytic establishment, their stated theories of mental health problems, which did not include any acknowledgment of the role of external or environmental stress, and their view of emotion as part of neurosis or the playing out of unconscious fantasies. To Bowlby, it was clear that the basis of such problems was in communication! He began to listen to some of his mentors who believed that to study the mind or behavior without seeing context, and especially a person's most important relationships, was like studying fish without acknowledging water. Take fish out of water and they look like a different animal altogether.

It is fair to say that he became obsessed with separateness and connection and how they determined the psychological development of a child. It is not hard to understand how he became sensitive to this issue and the deprivation that arises from a lack of emotional connection and support in childhood. He grew up in a family with distant parents, where his closest relationship was with his nursemaid, Minnie, who left the family when he was 4 years old. As an adult, he described this loss as

15

a "tragic" event and always kept Minnie's picture up in his bedroom. He was sent to English boarding school at the age of 10 and continued to see the results of emotional loss and isolation on children when he worked as a young adult at Priory Gate School and the London Child Guidance Clinic. During World War II, he protested at the evacuation of young children to the countryside without their families, citing a study that showed it was less damaging for children to be in danger from bombing in the cities than to be taken away from the emotional safety offered by their loved ones.

Bowlby believed in science, in testing ideas in the real world. After the war, he set up a research unit at the Tavistock Clinic and went on to systematically study the interactions between mothers and their children in detail. The mother-child drama he set up and studied was simple but profound. He observed what happens to a child in an unfamiliar situation when a mother leaves the room for a few minutes, how this induces a sense of alarm and helplessness in the child, and then what happens when she returns. How does the mother react to a child's distress, and how does the child deal with the threat of separation and renewed contact with a key attachment figure? Does the child panic on separation and become demanding and throw a tantrum on the mother's return? Do they shut down and look indifferent? Or does the child seek comfort and take it in when it is offered, finding emotional calm and balance? This drama that Bowlby construed reveals the essential secrets of who we are as human beings. It tells us how our nervous system responds to social connection or distance and how we are wired to deal with threat. It holds the secrets to the nature of love and why it matters so much, showing us what we need to grow and what constrains our ability to learn, thrive, and adapt to new situations.

Although he was hated and reviled as a heretic by many of his colleagues for years, Bowlby became one of the great pioneering geniuses of psychology and went on to found the theory and science of attachment and bonding. This theory states that we are essentially social bonding beings, always interdependent with others, and that emotional isolation is traumatizing in and of itself. Attachment theory is simply the most profound, most empirically tested understanding that has ever been constructed of personality and relationships and of how we develop our strengths and vulnerabilities. This makes it the ideal platform to grasp the chaos and pain of traumatic experience and to delineate a map to bringing healing and closure to that experience.

However, Bowlby mostly focused on the interaction between mothers and children. Such was the contempt for so called "dependency" in adulthood that it was not until the beginning of this century that it was acknowledged that attachment is not just about childhood, it operates in important ways from the cradle to the grave. The work on adult attachment did not begin to flower until around the year 2000, with the work of researchers such as Phillip Shaver and Mario Mikulincer. It was around then that a certain young clinical psychology professor was perhaps a part of this flowering (Johnson, 1986), when in a sudden golden moment of insight, I (Sue) realized that the pivotal moments of transformation she was seeing in a couple intervention called EFT (which she had just created and tested) were classic bonding events. In these bonding events, labeled *softenings,* partners became Accessible, Responsive, and emotionally Engaged (ARE) with each other. These are the exact responses that Bowlby found typified loving mothers who shaped a sense of security and confidence in their children. He had pinpointed the dance that defined secure love—parental and romantic. In EFT, this dance changed distressed relationships into positive, lasting bonds, and the bonding process also seemed to grow the dancers into more balanced, flexible, resilient people—just as Bowlby outlined it would. We are wired for connection with others. To be deprived of it has the same effects as being deprived of food or oxygen. The myth of the self-sufficient human fueled by so called drives like competitiveness, aggression, and sexuality is the most dangerous toxic lie any culture has ever come up with. As the primatologist Frans de Waal states, "We would not be here today had our ancestors been socially aloof." Caring and cooperating are key to survival.

The field of adult attachment has now flowered, at least in terms of studies and academic books (Johnson, 2019; Mikulincer & Shaver, 2023), and it has entered our communal awareness. We do not send our children off to the hospital alone for a week or so to be operated on by strangers, as was the norm 60 years ago. We allow partners into birthing rooms to hold women's hands because we know it reduces pain and panic. Conversely, researchers have started to take experiences like rejection by others seriously (Eisenberger et al., 2003; Eisenberger & Lieberman, 2004; Johnson, 2013), finding that when we are excluded or ignored, even by peers rather than attachment figures, this registers in the anterior cingulate cortex (ACC), the same part of the brain that registers physical pain.

Like us, other clinicians have published brain scan research. Ours showed that after bonding conversations, holding a partner's hand neutralizes in the brain the impact of the threat of electric shock (Johnson et al., 2013). A secure sense of connection to a close other is the primary "solution" to fear and vulnerability for our species. Slowly, even in a society addicted to a focus on the self, we are getting Bowlby's message. It has been slow to permeate the field of mental health and intervention, however. A few models of therapy give a passing nod to attachment science, and some are now beginning to integrate it more formally, but we know of none except ourselves who have studied bonding responses and their impact and used attachment as a wholistic way of understanding and healing our fellow humans—and of course, ourselves.

SO WHAT DOES ALL THIS SCIENCE SAY EXACTLY?

Maybe before setting out the principles supporting this work, we need to first lay out some of the core concepts about just who we are as humans.

Firstly, like clinicians such as Carl Rogers, attachment science privileges emotion as the key organizer of the most significant parts of our inner life and of our primary relationships. The attachment perspective states that emotion compellingly focuses our attention on what matters most to us in the stream of perception and experience. Emotion communicates to our inner selves, and to others, key messages concerning our deepest needs, our survival concerns. It acts like a compass, telling us where we are and motivating us—turning us toward specific actions, such as angry protest at being rejected. This contrasts with the popular view that emotions are unreasonable, random, somehow a source of weakness and not to be trusted. Emotions have been called by some, like Hobart Mowrer (1960), a higher order of intelligence. Once you have a map to our emotional life, every emotional response emerges as perfectly reasonable. We will talk more about emotion in Chapter 3, when we outline how attachment science guides healing. Emotional health is about having access to one's feelings, being able to tune into and explore them, and keeping one's emotional balance in a manner that allows distress to be framed as manageable and the self to be viewed as worthy and competent. As stated in the book *Love Sense* (Johnson, 2013), "Emotion is a sharp smart force that organizes and enlivens our lives. It is what transforms existence into experience." The painter Henri Matisse said, "I do not literally paint the table but the emotion it produces upon me." Good relationships with parents, partners, or professional helpers are ones where we feel seen and accepted and are empathized with, so that our emotions become clearer and more coherent. In such relationships, emotions themselves become more known, less frightening, more acceptable and manageable. They can then be used as a source of growth—as a way to come home to ourselves.

The second key concept that underpins the attachment frame, namely that we are relational beings always interdependent with others, is both simple and huge in its implications. Our need for emotional connection with others has shaped our neural architecture, our responses to stress, our emotional lives, and the interpersonal dramas and dilemmas that make up those lives. Our young are ridiculously vulnerable for longer than any other species. Without constant attention and care, they die. In order to survive, we had to join together, comfort and protect each other, hunt together, and refine our communication to shape cooperative groups. Constructive dependency on others is key to mental health and happiness. This perspective tells us that our sense of self, our model of who we are, is an ongoing construction, a process rather than an object, and one that is defined by interactions with others. Positive connection can heal us and help us thrive. Without this connection, we are like a plant without light, and if we are isolated and rejected, we feel our fragility in our very bones. For any healer, grandmother, physician, or therapist, this implies that showing up with explicit compassion and attunement is a key part of the healing process. If we expect wounded people to open up to us, then we must be willing to be authentic, engaged, and present with them, to send the signal that they are safe with us. We all tune into the level of engagement that is offered to us in an interaction.

The third key point is that true healing is more than coping, problem-solving, or reducing symptoms; it is about helping a person expand into a stronger, more grounded sense of self, deepening their awareness and connection with themselves and probing the places where they are stuck, frozen in distress. In this frozen state, they are unable to explore their experience, caught in panicking and chaotic catastrophizing or rigid shutting down and numbing out. Attachment is a developmental model of how the personality grows across time, and how that growth is fostered or hindered especially by the key dramas and relationships in a person's life. It is a therapist's job then, to believe in their client's potential and to find and explicate this person's strengths, even when their behavior is less than positive. The goal in an attachment-oriented therapy is that each client has access to a secure connection with self and with key others. We ask others, most often only with implicit cues, "ARE you there for me?" as in, "A: accessible and open to me; R: responsive to me; and E: emotionally engaged with me so that I feel valued and important." In terms of a secure connection with a sense of self, most trauma survivors say things such as:

"I have lost myself—I don't know who I am."
"Maybe I am defective, and I should have been able to prevent what happened."
"I shut down so I can't feel me anymore. I am just a ghost."
"I don't want to know, to see what is inside me."
"I can't see the face of me as a small child—it's a blank."
"When I think of my trauma, I just tell myself how weak I am and how I should have known better."

"I don't know what you mean. How can I feel bad for that weak part of me?"

"I deserve to suffer for what I did."

"I just spend my life getting mad at people or numbing out and drinking or stuffing food in my mouth."

"I don't think I can talk like this—this is way too close to things that churn my stomach, and you are too chummy for me."

Nowhere in these statements do you find what research tells us is typical of secure connection with self and others, namely, an ability to tune into and name the flow of experience; a confidence in one's ability to manage distress in this flow; a trust that this emotionally loaded experience is valid and can be trusted; and a trust in closeness with others. Particularly relevant for those who are traumatized and so especially sensitive to failure of any kind, is that more secure children tend to respond to potential failure and risk with increased effort, whereas those who are less secure often respond with helplessness and defeatism (Lutkenhaus et al., 1985). Healers can be hopeful that once secure connection is primed and experienced, it tends to be self-reinforcing, recognized by every neuron in our body as a source of joy and the answer to our deepest longings.

Finally, attachment science provides us with a framework for understanding the core structure of our shared humanity. That is, our hard-wired, psychobiologically based attachment systems; our need for belonging and connection, the role of emotion as a central organizer of self and experience, and the finite number of ways we have for managing stress and distress. We recognize, as well, that the way these central underlying features of attachment are expressed and manifested will vary across groups, communities, and cultures, even within the same family or person across time and relationship. This is evident, for example, in the variation of emotional expression, as well as the meaning of emotion in different contexts (e.g., see Guillory, 2022; Mesquita, 2022; Mesquita & Walker, 2002). Noteworthy as well and increasingly studied are the implications of identity in relationship, as well as the intersection between identity and context, including the therapeutic relationship (e.g., see Petty-John et al., 2020). The importance of mental health professionals adapting therapeutic interventions to meet the unique and diverse contextual and cultural realities of their clients has also been highlighted (e.g., see Allan et al., 2022; Davis et al., 2018; Hayes & Allan, 2024; Karakurt & Keiley, 2009; Linhoff & Allan, 2019; Nightingale et al., 2019). With this in mind and recognizing that the research literature is likely lagging behind the social and cultural realities of many of our clients, we wish to emphasize the importance of joining with each client from a place of curiosity, not assumption, and with a stance of humility. The attachment lens is intended to be held in a manner that affords breadth and depth, with a recognition of the central influence of context on past, present, and future, on the manifestation and expression of emotion, and on an ever-evolving sense of self in relationship. This is discussed further in later chapters where we highlight the importance of attending to context, attachment, the therapeutic alliance, and emotion at therapy outset and throughout the therapy process.

THE FOUR PRINCIPLES OF ATTACHMENT

Safe haven connection is the first of four principles of attachment. The foremost conclusion of the thousands of studies on human attachment is that safe human connection is THE evolutionary niche where humans do not just survive, they thrive, learn, and grow. This is not about companionship or social connection, per se, it is about emotional connection with someone you trust who offers you comfort—a safe haven when you are vulnerable. A felt sense of this connection is a primary need; it is coded by our nervous system as a matter of survival. For children, this connection has to be tangible; they need to be physically touched and held. For adults, this sense of connection can be triggered by an emotionally laden image held in the mind. For some adults, this can be a sense of connection with a spiritual figure. In a safe-haven relationship, you know that you matter to this other person. You know that they feel with you and for you, that you are valued by them, and that you can count on them to come when you call. This internal recognition turns distress into something tolerable and manageable and offers the possibility of emotional balance. In our form of therapy for distressed couples, we watched hundreds of couples find the way to becoming emotionally open and responsive to each other. We documented the positive effects of this new safe-haven connection on their relationships, on anxiety, on depression and traumatic stress, and on each partner's sense of competence and confidence. Conversely, we found that emotional isolation induces helplessness and emptiness (Holt-Lunstad et al., 2015).

A common phrase in Latin and also used by a shaman porcupine in Sue's first work of fiction, *Edgar & Elouise* (Johnson, 2022), "Ipso facto, there it is.": To stare the monster that is trauma in the face, name it and tame it, we need a sense of safe-haven connection, to know that there is someone who stands with us. To stand alone most often induces paralysis or panic. In mental health settings, a sense of safe haven can be provided by an attuned therapist who is emotionally available and responsive, that is, if the therapist knows how to shape this kind of safety. In such a haven, we can allow our longings and softer feelings to arise, risk reaching for another and clearly express our needs to them, and take in the care that is given, finding our balance and strength. These actions are foreign for many, especially those who have been abused and traumatized by attachment figures. A natural mistrust and reluctance to let down one's guard makes a sense of safe haven at once more crucial and more difficult to achieve.

A *secure base* is the second principle of attachment. Once we have the balance conferred by a sense of safe haven, we find that we also have a secure base for exploration and risk taking. It makes all the difference when someone has our back. Emotional connection and effective dependency, where we know how to access and can expect the support of others, make us stronger, more able to deal with threat and uncertainty. It is the child whose parent stays engaged, smiles, names the fear and reassures, who climbs up the ladder and lets their body explode down the slide. They reach the ground feeling competent and clever. It is the young businesswoman who acknowledges her fears and seeks support by confiding in her partner, who expresses less self-doubt, takes more risks, and rises faster in her profession (Feeney, 2004). There are many studies revealing that the victims of war and of childhood physical and sexual abuse who have an inner sense of safe attachment and supportive relationships with others show less PTSD symptoms and are more able to heal after such traumas (Mikulincer et al., 1993).

Even simply priming with attachment-oriented words, such as "being loved," that flash up on a screen so fast that people cannot consciously register them, reduces reactivity and terror responses to real-life threats such as being bombarded in war (Mikulincer et al., 2006). A therapist feels good when a client like Amy tells her, "You get it, don't you? You are not afraid of my pain. You seem to feel like I can deal with this, open up to this—you tell me I can. And I feel like you are with me here and you know where we are going. Do you know where we are going with all this?" It is important that the therapist can reply with a confident affirmation.

Accessibility, Responsiveness and Engagement (ARE) is the third concept that is central to the attachment perspective. That is, *accessibility*, sensitive empathic *responsiveness,* and emotional presence or *engagement* shape a sense of security in others. When this is our usual way of being, then we can also be self aware and open to our own more vulnerable selves, responding with self-compassion and care. What attachment figures model in patterns of emotionally charged interactions we then internalize and use as a way of relating to ourselves. Even the most wounded are often able to find their way to a safe haven and secure base if given on target attachment-oriented responses.

In contrast, when we experience or are threatened with rejection or abandonment from those we turn to, this triggers a wired-in response pattern of protest (which often looks simply like anger or hostile demands), then of panic and despair, and finally numbing and detachment. If this rejection is chronic, an inability to trust others or one's own longings for connection sets in and isolation is all that remains. This delineation of emotional pattern is just part of the map to our emotional life that attachment science offers us. The map allows us to see past surface reactions to someone's core reality—their heartscape.

  The ability to explore and learn is the fourth principle of attachment. Belonging and the safety it offers us leads to the ability to explore and learn—to become. Attachment science has shown that people program their mental models of who they are and what to expect from others from the repetitive dramas played out with those closest to them. These models are often referred to as styles and include protocols, the if-this-then-that understanding of how to respond to our own needs and emotions and how to interact with others. They become automatic and unconscious responses and can bias how we perceive ongoing events. Why do I (Sue) flip into icy hostility when someone defines me in a negative way? It is a direct feedback loop to my old dance pattern with my mother, who was so worried that her daughter might get what she called a "swelled head" that she delivered a steady stream of negative criticism. Now, decades later, this dance can still take me over—unless I catch it first and step aside! More security goes along with a more positive sense of self and a more forgiving response to inevitable failures and mistakes. In fact, a sense of security is associated with every kind of positive variable connected to mental health and positive functioning. Securely attached people are better at seeking support, taking it in and using it, and giving it to others. They are more empathic and assertive, more flexible when problem solving, and of course, more effective in terms of affect regulation. In the catastrophe of 9/11, it was the securely attached survivors who did not experience PTSD and were more likely to find their way to growth and resilience (Fraley et al., 2006).

  When we are deprived or traumatized and cannot find any safe connection with self or with others, then our most adaptive primary secure strategy is very difficult to access. When that happens, our emotional regulation options are limited. We turn to more insecure options, called secondary strategies or styles, that consist of either ramping up arousal in what is usually called "anxious preoccupied attachment," or dampening this arousal in "avoidant dismissing attachment." Like the secure style, these are not absolutes; they exist on a continuum, and we usually develop a primary style and then a backup. Both these secondary strategies begin as ways to protect the self from chaos and negative interactions with key others, but if allowed to become rigid and generalized, then they limit our mental and emotional perceptions and responses. Both the anxious preoccupied and the anxious avoidant strategies have been linked to higher levels of depression, anxiety, and traumatic stress, but avoidance is also associated with substance abuse and antisocial problems. Both strategies negatively impact the creation of positive attachment relationships in adulthood and so inhibit the creation of healing emotional connection.

Anxious attachment, found in research studies to arise from unpredictable or insensitive parenting and early separation from attachment figures, is characterized by a preoccupation with reassuring connection to others, a sensitivity to any perceived abandonment and rejection, as well as cognitive responses like catastrophizing. Sunita tells me, "If I am going out to meet friends from work, I plan every move, every statement. I know it will all go wrong. Then I can't pull the plan off. I end up withdrawing and numbing, so people ignore me, and I go home more alone than ever. I can't sleep and then the ghosts come and devour me, like they did when I was small. My mum used to get so angry if I woke her when I so, so carefully tried to climb into her bed at night. I can't sleep with the light off even now." Anxious adults in distressed relationships often appear angry and demanding, but if you really listen, they are protesting disconnection, sending distorted attachment signals. They are asking, "Where are you—are you there for me?" Tragically, their angry surface emotional expression makes it harder for their partners to respond, and they set up the blame/withdraw cycles that predict marriage breakdown.

Avoidant attachment typically develops when support figures are emotionally absent or indifferent or actively dangerous. The child has little choice but to shut down and try to freeze all vulnerabilities and all unmet longings for connection, distracting themselves with toys, tasks, and activities. As adults, they have a great reluctance to open up to their own emotions or acknowledge any need for connection. They do not want to count on others in any way. This kind of need is viewed as a defect or weakness. We learn that what is not responded to when we are young and most vulnerable is best not seen or named. When, after 20 years of marriage, Aiyana tearily tells Dakari in my office that she is so lonely that she has decided she cannot reach him and has no choice but to leave him, Dakari sits stone faced and quietly replies, "Fine. If that is what you want." Aiyana leaves him and Dakari falls apart, asking me what is wrong with him; why has he turned into "a pathetic wimp." Avoidance is a fragile strategy in the end. Our needs and wired-in longings are not so easily dismissed. Saul, a war vet, tells me, "I don't ever remember being held or feeling close growing up. I can't tell you what I feel. It's not my thing. I play my video games and exercise. But everything is meaningless—like empty. Not sure why I don't just put a gun to my head. Once in a while, I get really, really mad, that is all."

There is just one more insecure option besides falling into perpetual anxiety or shutting down, which is simply to do both in turn. This has, for obvious reasons, been called disorganized attachment. These clients are often labeled "borderline" or "simply crazy." However, this flipping between hyperarousal and hypoarousal, between panic and detachment, is a logical life strategy when we note the specific circumstances where this strategy was learned and was, perhaps, the only way to survive. Disorganized attachment is rooted in early experience where caretakers—the potential sources of safety, comfort, and protection—who are desperately needed in threatening situations, are, at the same time, also the source of terror and pain. This constitutes a "violation of human connection" (Herman, 1992) that has huge existential and mind scrambling consequences. The difference between love and abuse is often scrambled and impossible for a child to comprehend. Children and adults who have been sexually and physically traumatized by family members often display this strategy and are particularly vulnerable to being retraumatized as adults and to experiencing PTSD. In relationships, they flip between frantic demanding and vigilance for any signs of nonresponsiveness, coupled with an inability to trust that then triggers distancing and disassociation. We should note that once we put this paradoxical style and seemingly irrational behavior in the context of attachment, where close others are desperately needed AND also desperately dangerous, it all makes exquisite sense. So, I can say to Mary Ellen, "Of course you want to angrily scream at your partner when I ask you to close your eyes and picture him right now. You want to say, 'Can't you see how hurt and scared I am. I need you to comfort me, not give me reasons and explanations.' At the same time, when we imagine him responding gently to you, you go very still, move into a 'fog.' Of course. You are desperate for comfort and terrified to trust it and take it in." Mary Ellen looks at me with tears in her eyes and whispers, "I have no place to put it. And it's not for me—for someone like me." As she allows and names her pain and her pattern, she allows herself to grieve and accept the "crazy" survival strategy that is now imprisoning her. Using an attachment frame allows us to see the logic in this kind of behavior and to dissolve the shame that Mary Ellen feels. Isolation burns and so does risking and needing, colored by terror and betrayal.

There was a time when theorists believed that once these ways of relating to ourselves, our emotions, and to others were set in attachment patterns that became consolidated in our cognitive models of self and others, they simply played out across the lifespan. Now we know that is not true. As with most emotionally loaded factors defining our early life, while they echo forward so that there is some stability across time, change is also possible. Key traumas or betrayals inflicted by loved ones, as well as positive experiences of secure connection, can transform us. Children can move into insecure patterns when their parents divorce. Adults can move from a secure model of self and other into these insecure patterns when they become caught in an abusive romantic relationship, where the friend and comforter is also the enemy. In one of our most significant studies on EFT for distressed couples (Johnson et al., 2013), we showed that bonding conversations where previously distressed partners were guided to share vulnerability, reaching and responding to each other's attachment needs, partners became more securely attached to each other. They were able to access their need for connection, send new, more coherent emotional messages, and display new levels of empathy and emotional engagement with others. If we understand attachment and know how to tap into attachment patterns, we can begin to change this key aspect of personality and relational life for the better. Once this way of dealing with emotions and defining the self changes, then more adaptive responses to traumatic experience and increased resilience come online.

PROVEN AND PROFOUND BUT DOWN TO EARTH

Attachment science is rich, profound, and empirically based, but it is also a very down-to-earth perspective. We can look at key responses in trauma survivors through an attachment lens and see into and order the everyday reactions of these survivors more clearly. Science is basically the discovery and elucidation of patterns, of self reinforcing recurring processes. What are some of the emotional and relational patterns common to trauma survivors that the attachment lens pinpoints and make sense of?

Attachment highlights and makes sense of the fact that without a grounded sense of belonging, continued emotional and relational development is constrained. It is almost impossible to really risk and explore and grow when we do not feel seen and safe. This emphasizes the need for safe connection in challenging moments that threaten our world, in close relationships, in mental health interventions, and in medical settings. This is especially crucial when our nervous system has been raked raw by trauma cues. The need for a safe therapeutic alliance is mentioned in almost every model of therapy but a real knowledge of exactly what such safety entails and how to shape it is often missing. Attachment offers us a clear model of what connection with a stronger, wiser other looks like and how it works. This will be discussed further, later in this book.

Even in therapies explicitly focused on improving a relationship between clients—couple therapy—the focus is more often on problem solving, communication skills, or sexual exploration, rather than the shaping of more secure connection. In our work with distressed couples dealing with the aftermath of trauma in one or more partners, we find that once emotional openness, responsiveness, and engagement are present, then communication and problem-solving skills can be accessed and used effectively. Safe ground allows us to engage fully and find more flexible solutions to almost any problem. First, of course, the therapist must create a safe haven with each client, even in the face of totally opposing perspectives that these clients might have. (There is an example of how to work with trauma in couple therapy later in this book.)

As previously stated, attachment tells us about our deepest longings for emotional connection and acceptance by key others, and just how crucial they are to our survival. It shows us how these longings can spur growth and wholeness; they motivate us to risk and to reach for new parts of ourselves and for others. However, they can also paradoxically be part of how we become trapped in responses like anxiety, denial, and the continual avoidance of trauma cues. For example, attachment theorists point out that a sense of connection, of mattering to another, is so compelling a need that people can find themselves appeasing and even protecting an abusive other. The logic behind this is that it is better to cling to a bad object than to have none at all (Fairbairn, 1952). Isolation terrifies us all. Malee has worked so hard, dealing with the echoes of abuse by her father, but she is still caught somehow. As her therapist explores her ongoing terror of abandonment and sense of aloneness, it suddenly becomes clear that the source of pain that is still being studiously avoided is her relationship with her mother, who saw but ignored the abuse, and now denies that it happened at all. This is the loss, the starvation, the "How could you?" and the "Wasn't I worth protecting?" that still haunts Malee's dreams. Research makes it clear that the deprivation of safe connection that keeps us constantly uncertain and at risk can be as toxic as other types of maltreatment such as physical or sexual abuse (e.g., see Teicher & Samson, 2016; Strathearn et al., 2020). The therapist validates that Malee's clinging to the idea that her mother was not part of her trauma allowed her to cling to a modicum of safety and find a way to survive in her darkest times, but it came with a price. Once Malee can experience and grieve her loss, she finds a new level of closure around her trauma and a new clarity as to what she needs in an adult relationship.

The understanding of the existential significance of our fears about abandonment and rejection and how they can leave us hanging in terrifying no-solution vulnerability makes sense of the negative moves we engage in to try to escape this pain. Very often trauma survivors would rather take things upon themselves and decide that they are to blame or deserved their trauma, rather than really acknowledge and accept the careless cruelty or indifference of key others and the complete sense of helplessness that accompanies this. Jeff is enveloped in shame, telling his therapist, "I am selfish, disgusting and pathetic. I tried to prove I was the son my father wanted and my mother longed for but . . . I let them down. So they were right to punish and shun me. If I had tried harder . . . " There is hope here but also continual despair because he is still failing to please and is caught in a web of longing, anguish, nightmares, and self-castigation. He cannot hear that, never having been seen or accepted for who he was, he now joins with his parents and treats himself the same way. He cannot, when asked, see the face of the small boy who was starved of connection and who turned himself inside out to please, but lost himself in the process. He denies his longing for acceptance and his rage, feeling only numbness or free-floating anger. Once the therapist can join him where he is and make sense of this, doors into the way he shapes his narrow, inner emotional world begin to open.

Attachment takes us past abstract labels that we or others place on ourselves. These labels can help us, but they also stigmatize. Recently, a diagnosis of ADHD in childhood was found to offer no improvement in factors like happiness in adolescence, and to, in fact, negatively impact self-efficacy and undermine a positive sense of self (Kazda et al., 2022). Labels are also so general that for the public and for professional helpers, they offer little guidance as to how to find the way out of the forest of problems like depression. Bowlby himself reminds us that depression is most often shorthand for "lonely, unlovable, unwanted, and helpless." In an attachment-oriented therapy where you learn to listen to yourself, identify different levels of your emotions, and experience another tuning into and grounding you, you find the specific reality behind the labels.

There are also times when an attachment focus actually allows us to label things more accurately as attachment injuries and recognize their impact.

Symptoms of distress, which as mentioned before are most often protective strategies that have become all encompassing and imprisoning, can also be seen as acceptable and logical when viewed from the compassionate attachment lens. The tendency to dissociate is often part of the diagnosis of PTSD, however, it can turn up very differently in different people and can also be viewed as a survival strategy when all else fails, rather than as pathological. For Harriet, it was once the only way out of nightmares and flashbacks, but blaming herself for this only keeps her caught on a treadmill of shame and ever-escalating distress. Once she accepts this much needed escape, she can step past it and gradually let herself confront the reality glimpsed in the flashback.

In short, the attachment map to core emotions, strategies for regulating them, and models of identity offers all of us an outline of the plot in the drama called being human. This means that we can:

- Recognize and tune into our own inner vulnerabilities and those of the people we wish to help.
- Order and accept these realities, seeing their universality and the part they play in survival.
- Regulate these emotional realities, see how we construct them, and explore their mental representations.
- Understand and reflect on our responses to ourselves and others, from both a micro moment-to-moment, specific, tangible level and a macro level, where we see what humanness entails and how very basically human we are.
- Use our new groundedness and secure base to shift emotions and models to shape growth and transformation. Emotions evoke new action tendencies.

Saul is finally able to "see" the face of his small, fragile self and naturally, his chest fills with a new emotion—compassion—and the ability to accept and comfort that small part of himself. His shame-based identity shifts into a recognition of his hunger for acceptance and the walls he puts up, risking opening up to others. Until this dilemma is resolved, he cannot move. His traumatic experience has him by the throat. Core emotions focus us on new versions of need and belonging, new realities where attempts to regulate "frightening, alien, and unacceptable emotion" no longer rule our life. The way to letting go of trauma—to reaching our own version of closure and completeness—is to walk this path. This is the most natural, wired-in process of healing. Our research results in so many studies and all our clients have taught us that most of us can do it—if we are guided by a trusted other and the path is made clear.

Finally, it is worth stating that we are living at a time when, as psychologist Jonathon Haidt (2023) describes it, "chaos, fragmentation and outrage seem to reign supreme." The world is divided into oppressors or victims and constant self censorship in the name of freedom is becoming the norm. It is also a time when loneliness and loss of social connection has been deemed a serious mental health problem. Many of us now look at screens and read texts, when we used to spend so much of each day looking into faces. The epidemic of depression and suicidality in our youth, which seems to have begun as the iPhone entered our lives, should concern us all (Haidt, 2023). In this context, it makes sense that it would be harder and harder for many of us to find the resilience that comes with an inner sense of safe haven and secure base, and to find the relationships that offer these essential experiences. It seems inevitable that more and more of us will be increasingly caught in the web of the many traumatic events that assail us. It is, then, even more crucial that we identify the core elements in healing and the best way to grow past apparently impossible challenges.

Therapy is not the only way to grow out of trauma, however, the ability of a competent therapist to tune into and move with a client as they discover and rediscover their inner and relational world offers an often unique and potent corrective experience. The therapy session offers the opportunity to go to the leading edge of experience and focus on the defining elements of that experience in a way that clients find absorbing, empowering, and transformational. New emotional music leads to a new dance, which leads to a new sense of self, a new dancer.

PLAY AND PRACTICE

For You Personally

What is your prototypical strategy for managing distress? At times of feeling overwhelmed, do you tend to turn emotion up or down, or some combination of both? What do you notice among your loved ones? What are their prototypical strategies and how do their reactions impact you? Write some notes and during a period of connection with a significant other, and as comfortable, have a conversation about your respective attachment strategies/styles.

For You Professionally

What is your current understanding of how trauma impacts adaptive functioning? How is it the same or different based on what you have read here about attachment science as a path to healing? Regardless of your preferred intervention up to now, is this a framework that fits for you as a means of understanding and beginning to join with your clients and their presenting problems? Again, write some notes and as comfortable, have a conversation with a peer or group of peers.

KEY TAKEAWAYS

Four Core Assumptions about Who We Are as Humans

1. Emotion is the key organizer of our inner lives and primary relationships.
2. We are wired for connection.
3. We all have the capacity to grow but can get stuck in chaotic, catastrophizing, reactive intensification of emotion or rigid shutting down and numbing out.
4. Although our expression of emotion, needs, fears, and longings vary significantly, the basic underlying positive or negative processes by which we cope with crises, deprivation, and trauma, are patterned and predictable.

Principles of Attachment

Safe connection with key others is the ecological niche in which humans learn, grow, and thrive.

Attachment provides a map that allows us to see past surface reactions to someone's core reality—their heartscape.

Emotional connection and effective dependency confer increased confidence, competence, and resilience.

A safe sense of belonging leads to becoming (i.e., an ever-evolving sense of self).

Attachment security can be seen on a continuum.

Attachment sets the tone but is not set in stone. As with most emotionally loaded factors defining our early life, while they echo forward and there is some stability across time, change is also possible.

How Does Attachment Science Make Sense of the Common Impacts of Trauma?

Constrained emotional and relational development is the natural consequence of a lack of safety and belonging.

Symptoms of distress are most often protective strategies that have become all-encompassing and imprisoning and are seen as logical when viewed through a compassionate attachment lens.

The existential significance of our fears about abandonment and rejection and how they can leave us hanging in terrifying, no-solution vulnerable moments help us make sense of the negative moves we engage in to try to escape this pain. It is better to blame ourselves than to acknowledge the careless cruelty or indifference of key others.

The attachment map to core emotions, strategies for regulating them, and models of identity offer an outline of the plot in the drama of what it means to be human. This means we can:

- Recognize and tune into the core vulnerabilities of ourselves and others.
- Regulate these emotional realities, understand their origins, and explore their mental representations.
- Understand and reflect on our responses and those of others at a moment-to-moment, highly specific, and tangible level, highlighting what being human really entails.
- Use a secure base as a resource to shift emotions and patterns of interaction to shape growth and transformation.
- Identify the core elements in healing and the best way to become resilient and grow past apparently impossible challenges, especially important during times of threat or pervasive loneliness and social isolation.

3

The Five EFT Macro Interventions

A better understanding of ourselves and of traumatic experience and how it can define us and reverberate in our lives is crucial. But it is not enough.

We know that trauma can result in what psychologists call *posttraumatic growth,* that is, a traumatizing event can be experienced as a challenge that has been overcome. The Posttraumatic Growth Inventory (PTGI; Tedeschi & Calhoun, 1995) asks people to rate their agreement with statements like, "I can handle difficulties," "I changed my priorities about what is important in life," "I more clearly see how I can count on people in times of trouble," and "I can better appreciate each day." However, for most of us, even if we manage to find some positives, to recover from trauma is a struggle, and for many it becomes a never-ending nightmare.

What we want is a way OUT—an escape. But escape attempts have a way of placing us on a treadmill, where symptoms just recur. What seems to work best is to find a way THROUGH, and many, at some point, turn to a therapist for help with that. The key issue for practitioners then, is to find solutions to the helplessness and despair that are part of the client's PTSD. We need solutions that get to the heart of the matter and transform the core of this distress, that is, the process of emotional hijacking and numbing, vigilant catastrophizing, avoidance, and the perspective on self as helpless, damaged, or deficient.

EFT integrates three threads into the tapestry that is a therapy session. These threads are:

1. Attachment science and the map to human function it provides.
2. A ramped up and refined version of the interventions outlined by Carl Rogers, who believed, like Bowlby, that empathic

relationships are healing, and that resilience and growth are our birthright.
3. The clinical knowledge gained from 35 years of practice and research on EFT as an effective model of intervention.

The set of five macro interventions, what we call the EFT Tango, are the guide for the way THROUGH and the solution that we have found works best for the emotional dysregulation that so commonly characterizes the impacts of trauma (Wiebe et al., 2025). This set of five "moves" is used across all three stages and modalities of emotionally focused therapy: EFIT, EFCT, EFFT—individual, couple, and family therapy.

This set of macro interventions combines all the basic therapy micro interventions, described in the next chapter, into a structured whole that leads reliably to the corrective emotional experiences that predict positive outcome after therapy and at follow-up on many significant variables. For example, more secure attachment and the coherent positive sense of self inherent in this attachment style; less depression, anxiety, and trauma symptoms such as dissociation; more relationship satisfaction and trust in others; and the ability to regulate difficult emotions.

WHY IS THIS SET OF FIVE MOVES CALLED THE EFT TANGO?

The name of the dance, *tango*, is a metaphor designed to capture the nature of the healing interventions and moments created in EFT, and indeed, offers insights into safe, positive, close relationships outside of the therapy room. Argentine tango is, for those who know its magic, the ultimate dance of attunement and finding synchrony with another. The emotional music structures the dance and two people are able to move as one. It is all about sensitive honed responsiveness. Synchrony holds a natural magic for our nervous system; moving together with someone seems to cast a spell over us—we are absorbed, intoxicated even. Bonding animals move together, in tune with each other, in mating rituals. Mothers and infants sense each other's inner state and level of arousal and respond in kind. This connection is also deeply fulfilling in and of itself. Each moment is a safe adventure, an unfolding.

The EFT Tango has five moves:

1. *Reflecting Present Process:* Outlining the process of how inner experience and interactions with others form into self-regenerating patterns that impact emotional balance, posttraumatic symptoms, and models of self and other.

2. *Assembling and Deepening Emotion:* Accessing the structure of emotional experience to befriend emotion, rendering it ordered, manageable, and acceptable. Emotion is then deepened to access vulnerabilities and longings that spur new actions.
3. *Choreographing Engaged Encounters:* Setting up a new way of relating to—a new dance with—key parts of oneself and with important others. These dramas epitomize the existential dilemmas at the heart of the client's struggles.
4. *Processing the Encounter:* Reflecting on and integrating the process of moves 2 and 3, particularly in terms of key shifts in emotion and the client's sense of self.
5. *Integrating and Validating:* Summarizing the above process in a manner that frames the client as competent, worthy, and able to grow.

These moves are reflected in Figure 3.1.

We can simplify things and turn this change process into the language of everyday life. Jim shifts to a metalevel of conversation and

Dancing THE
EFT TANGO

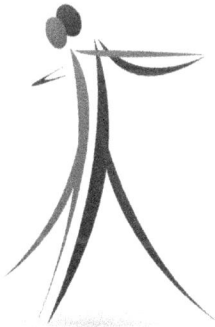

THE
5 BASIC
MOVES
OF EFT

1.
MIRRORING/
REFLECTING
PRESENT
PROCESS

2.
AFFECT
ASSEMBLY &
DEEPENING
(using the Elements of Emotion)

3.
CHOREO-
GRAPHING
ENGAGED
ENCOUNTERS

4.
PROCESSING
THE
ENCOUNTER

5.
INTEGRATING
&
VALIDATING

Elements
of Emotion:
› Trigger
› Perception
› Body
› Meaning
› Action

The second figure can be:
- a therapist
- an aspect of self
- an imaginary other in individual therapy
- a partner in couple therapy
- different family members in family therapy

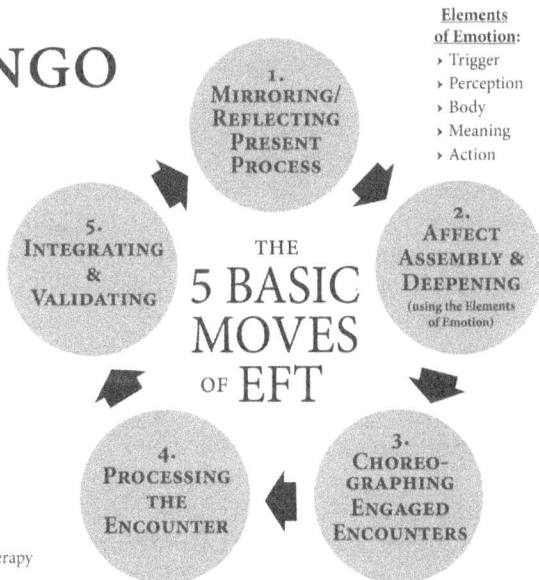

FIGURE 3.1. Dancing the EFT Tango—the five basic moves of EFT.

decides to talk about how he and Pete relate, instead of staying with informational content. Jim says to his best friend, Pete, "You know, you and I used to talk in a different way—a closer way. I could really open up to you. But now I somehow end up feeling guarded and less relaxed. And you seem more distant, too. I share less and then you seem to do the same—share less personal stuff. We end up talking about the weather, like we are doing now" (Move 1). "Last time we met I realized that I felt real tense when I left and sort of sad even. It felt like something was missing, but I told myself 'things change' so 'nothing to do here.' I sort of gave up on us. But now I realize that I do feel sad and I long for the closeness we used to have" (Move 2). Pete reflects what he is hearing in a soft voice and leans closer to Jim, asking him how long he has felt this way. Jim goes on, "Not sure. I guess I feel like I have lost you, somehow, as a real friend and that scares me. I guess I depend on our friendship and need to know it's still there. I would like us to reconnect" (Move 3). Pete echoes Jim's sentiments and says that he has been stressed and shut down but appreciates when Jim shares like this and reaches for him (Move 4). Jim says he really appreciates Pete being open and listening, and that he feels really good about himself, taking this risk and opening up this conversation. Jim and Pete smile as they drink their beer. This conversation changes their relationship and communicates to them both about what they need and who they are.

Therapy is the deliberate, intentional, and intensified version of a natural connection and growth process. The process here was characterized by ARE—Accessibility, Responsiveness, and Engagement—and the level of conversation shifted from a stand back metalevel to a deeper, more emotional level, and then to a balanced, integrating level. It takes awareness and a decision to stay focused and authentic.

It is important to stress that the EFT Tango is not a mechanical formula or a list to be invariably followed in a set order. It can be implemented at varying levels of intensity across stages and sessions. It is a metaphor that captures an alive, moving process of growth.

As seen in the *Primer for EFIT* (Johnson & Campbell, 2022), Henny was so thoroughly traumatized, dealing with the life crisis of separating from her addicted partner of many years and with echoes of extreme abuse in her childhood, that the first eight to nine sessions were spent building an alliance and trying to get a clear storyline of her chaotic version of her present and past life and her coping mechanisms. Whole sessions were spent in Move 1 of the Tango, trying to find clear patterns in her life and resource her for the journey of therapy. Conversely, Sunita, a highly anxious young woman with an eating disorder, was able to walk with the therapist in a light but focused way through all five moves of the Tango in the first session. Some sessions will mainly focus on just two moves in the Tango, for example in the process of Move 2 (Deepening Emotion) and Move 3 (Choreographing Engaged Encounters), reported in detail in a key Stage 2 session with Henny where she goes through a potent corrective emotional epiphany. In this session, she comforts her 8-year-old self after the first vicious rape by her father and deeply engages, for the first time, with the core emotions associated with this newly accessed memory. A micro intervention like validation will be interspersed throughout an EFIT session but is often used at the end of a session in a more extended and deliberate Move 5 manner to summarize and validate the positive steps the client has taken toward healing in the session.

EXPLORING THE MOVES OF THE EFT TANGO

Let's look at the five Tango moves in more detail. It is best to start with the preparation for embarking on the Tango in therapy. The therapist listens to clients' stories, follows and reflects the emotions in those stories, and notes how clients are showing up in the here and now, focusing on both vulnerabilities and strengths. From the beginning, the therapist is at once exploring and evoking, as well as holding and ordering, distressing experience. The therapist remembers that the overall goal is to turn what is frightening, alien, and unacceptable into what is manageable, normal, and an accepted part of self; that is, to shape a secure connection to a new sense of self that is competent and confident, and able to be trusted. The EFIT therapist expects that vigilance and catastrophizing will become curiosity and calm.

Preparation for the Tango

From the first moment of contact, the therapist attempts to:

- Send attuned safe haven signals, displaying a positive presence and sending signs typical of a surrogate attachment figure. This message sounds like, "I see you, hear you," "You are safe with me," "I am with you," and "We can order and deal with this together."
- Tune into key moments/pivotal experiences that have shaped affect regulation, views of self and other, and present protective strategies, such as dissociation or angry denial.
- Reflect both suffering and coping strategies, finding the logic in symptoms and difficulties, and unpacking abstract symptom labels.

- Reach for competence in each client, setting up expectations for success.
- Shape expectations for the therapy process, getting the client used to the way the therapist responds, for example, returning to and prioritizing emotion and the focus on present poignant experiencing.

The process of assessment, which is ongoing in EFIT and not only the beginning stage of therapy, is outlined and illustrated in a case description in a later chapter.

We will now examine in more detail the moves of the EFIT Tango and how the therapist intervenes in each move.

Move 1—Reflecting Present Processes

The therapist focuses on the dance with self and with key others. At first, focusing on the self of the client, the therapist:

- Reflects the client's present experience and past history, as well as how the client's past seems to be mirrored in the present. The focus is on patterns in the dance with the self. For example, does the client castigate and reprimand themselves or give up on themselves when they feel as if they have failed, and how do patterns of emotional regulation shape ongoing distress?
- Asks curious, evocative questions about emotions and explores how they are dealt with, discovering the ways clients relate to and construct their experience and themselves.
- Constantly pieces together the client's story of distress and their responses in a way that makes them coherent, logical, and understandable, finding key incidents in the past and present that resonate and confirm the story.
- Specifies and returns to the client's goal and longings in each therapy session. The focus here is on the question, "What does this client long for and what do they need?"

Also focusing on connections with others, the therapist:

- Reflects and asks evocative questions: the *how, what, when, where,* of key relationships and how these relationships impact the client. For example, asking a client, "What happens to you right now as we talk about your father and his terrifying violence?"
- Pieces together how client's and other's emotional signals organize

relationship dramas and how these dramas, in an exquisite, structured feedback loop, organize emotional responses and the connection with self. Inner and between realities loop together into a chain reaction—a recurring cycle.

• Paints a picture for the client in simple, evocative terms of the emotional music and dance steps with self and others that generate symptoms/problems and keep the client STUCK and unable to grow.

This is the heart of Move 1. The *process* of emotion regulation learned in dangerous and toxic places and the interpersonal responses that accompany it are the problem and block new perspectives and responses. They are the trauma trap that the client cannot exit from.

Example: "So, your relationship with your dad really created the defining drama in your life. He was so dangerous that the only safety was in being immediately accommodating or ready to totally 'disappear' as you put it, 'space out.' You never felt seen or held—this was alien—just did not seem to be for you? And even now with your partner, you always 'roll with everything' or just 'exit' where you don't even remember what happens from one day to the next. And the more you 'roll' or 'space out', the more lonely and 'small' you feel and the more he ignores you. So, you get more depressed and more spaced out to the point where you tell me that you 'don't know who you are'—your life is 'empty.' Do I have it right? But the only dance you know is to try to please or to 'disappear.' This leaves you more and more depressed and hopeless, yes?"

The desired outcome is that clients feel not only understood, but that a reliable, wiser other grasps a whole and coherent picture of the key elements of their problem, and it is not what they fear, which is that they are doomed, defective, and deficient. They are held and responded to as human beings stuck on the huge confusing wheel of life. As the therapist begins to outline the order and the recurring patterns of their experience, they begin to perceive their problems in a new way. Tara says to her therapist at the end of the first session, after sharing reams of detailed content descriptions of her different "hopeless" problems, "You get it." Finding the patterns and how they merge to shape a life, clarifies that life as well as its possibilities.

Move 2—Affect Assembly and Deepening (Using the Elements of Emotion)

In Move 2, the therapist focuses on and tracks emotion in present session in the process patterns of emotional regulation or interactional stories.

The aim is to look past the surface or acknowledged emotion to deeper, less owned emotion (e.g., past irritation to worry or fear). In EFT we think of emotion as a process, not a fact or finished product.

The therapist:

• Focuses on and tracks emotion, especially more primary emotional responses, in the present session and in the process patterns of emotion regulation or interactional stories. The therapist looks past the surface expressions of acknowledged affect to deeper, less explicit, less owned emotion (e.g., past irritation to worry and fear). Emotion is thought of as a process not a finished product. Example: "Can we stop a minute. You used the word 'irritated' again, but as you say it, you rub your hands together hard and look from side to side—almost like there is something scary happening here, some kind of threat, yes?" or, "You speak of being angry, but your face looks so still and kind of sad right now."

• Assembles the *elements of emotion*: trigger, basic first perception, body response, meaning making, and motivating action tendency. This process begins with first finding the specific trigger for the frightening, alien, and unacceptable feeling that the client is bypassing or cannot pinpoint. The map to affect used in EFIT outlines that there are six core emotional states that can be universally recognized and carry the same meaning across cultures: anger, joy, surprise, sadness, shame, and fear. Almost always, the last three listed are the underlying music behind guarded or fragmented surface expressions. The therapist accepts the surface response that the client offers but begins to explore by specifying when this emotion arises. The trigger is often viewed as a definition of the self of the client. Example:

THERAPIST: So, what was happening this morning when this vague bad feeling, or what you call "irritation" just came over you? You said your boss called you just before, and he was "pleasant."

CLIENT: Nothing happened. It's just my hormones. He wasn't mean. I just don't like talking to him.

THERAPIST: You don't like . . . could you help me understand a little more?

CLIENT: Um . . . I think it's his voice.

THERAPIST: What do you hear in his voice?

CLIENT: He doesn't think much of me. He thinks I am stupid. He doesn't care if I struggle with the impossible tasks he gives me. But it's fine—I don't mind really. No point in talking about it. Well, it's a bad scene. [The client's basic perception.]

THERAPIST: So you hear criticism and indifference in his voice. Like you are stupid and don't matter at all?

CLIENT: Yes. He's just like everyone else. My family specializes in indifference.

• Finds the specific *body sensation* that goes with the trigger, using very simple questions, mostly *what, where,* and *how* questions, and stays with and makes sensations vivid and specific. The therapist links the body experience to the trigger and repeats the link, as shown in the following example.

THERAPIST: So, you talk about irritation but, right now, as you talk about your boss's dismissal of you and your struggles, what happens inside your body?

This can be pressure, pain, heat, cold, constriction, movement, etc.: If the client says, "I don't know," then the therapist repeats the trigger and the question, and can also make conjectures, such as, "Perhaps you feel tight in your chest or . . . ?"

CLIENT: I feel shaky.

THERAPIST: Where do you feel this shaky feeling?

CLIENT: Right here—in my chest. I am kind of breathless.

• Finds the cognition/*meaning* that accompanies the trigger and the sensation; the way the client makes emotional meaning. This meaning is most often about the self, but it can be about others or life in general. Example:

THERAPIST: What do you say to yourself as this occurs?

CLIENT: I am invisible. No one sees me. I don't matter. Life is meaningless. It's not such a big deal. Maybe it was my fault.

• Reflects and repeats the trigger, sensation, and meaning, slowly and softly, making sense of this process in terms of the client's life story. The therapist validates and accepts this experience and the conclusions the client draws from it. As this enfolds, the client enters into the inquiry and moves into the felt sense of their experience, exploring it further. Deeper levels of emotion then become available. You may ask if this seems like one of the terrible trinity: sadness and grief; fear in its many forms; or shame. If empathically supported, the client will most often find their own heartfelt words here. Isolation, helplessness and no-solution, overwhelming vulnerability become apparent.

- Finds the *action impulse* that this emotional experience elicits. What do clients *do* in their everyday life when this emotion arises? What do they want to do here and now, as they feel this? Example:

THERAPIST: And when this happens, what do you want to do—what do you do?

CLIENT: I want to run. I shut down; I go into a fog; I shut people out; I get real down, down, down. There is nothing else to do.

- Integrates all the elements of emotion, putting the discovered trigger, perception, body sensation, cognition, and action impulse all together. The therapist reflects and repeats this integration several times so that the client can taste and absorb it. The therapist links this emotional process to the client's symptoms, problems, and views of self, asking for the client's input into the summary. The perspective on the basic pattern of emotional processing cursorily outlined in Move 1 now becomes more tangible and specific and begins to deepen. Example:

THERAPIST: So, when your boss calls, it's a "bad" situation and you get mad. But if you really feel it, there is a shakiness—you feel vulnerable, yes? And you say to yourself, "I am invisible, my feelings don't matter." This is so right in terms of how alone you were when you were being abused as a child—it makes sense. No one saw you, did they? So, you learned to shut down and now you tell yourself you are "depressed" and in that shut down, you shut everyone out—even the partner who loves you. Is this right? Help me correct it. And the more this circle spins, the more "depressed" you feel and the more shut down and empty. And you are once again, all alone.

The client may add to this overview by moving into common universal existential fears and dilemmas about isolation and rejection, meaninglessness and unmanageable vulnerability. The client might say, "My life is meaningless, empty; I am just defective, unlovable, sick. This will never change." Dilemmas emerge such as a longing to be seen and loved versus the desire to hide and not be seen and so be more vulnerable.

The therapist develops a shallow, reactive, vague labeling of emotion into specific, concrete, felt experience with this affect assembly. This experience can then be deepened further with techniques suggested previously, such as repetition, especially of poignant words or phrases that the client offers, the *emotional handles,* compelling imagery and metaphors that capture the client's reality, and speaking the music of safety by using a soft, slow prosody.

As a footnote to reflecting on Move 2, it might be useful to recap some of the most useful perspectives on emotion itself. Emotion *colors perception and meaning making* and *communicates* to us, as well as to others, our survival-oriented states and needs; it also *motivates* us, shifting our bodies and minds into action readiness (Johnson, 2019). As clients find new emotional realities and a new way to relate to emotion, all these ways of seeing and ordering experience, engaging with self and others, and action responses, begin to change. *Nothing rapidly reorganizes us and our world like core emotion.* Clients can benefit from cognitive skills focused on emotion regulation, insight, and sometimes even simple expression, although catharsis is not a useful concept from an EFT point of view, which focuses on restructuring emotion and emotional regulation to dramatically shift our habitual ways of being. An EFT therapist befriends, follows, and returns to emotion in session, much like following a musical theme. The clinician also shapes this music, making it louder or deeper, delving into it or repeating it. As mentioned earlier, poetry and plays, novels and musical events reflect this reality. Who can listen to the violinist Itzhak Perlman playing the theme from the movie *Schindler's List* without feeling the beginning of heartbreak? For the trauma survivor, this emotion goes straight to the heart of the matter.

Move 3—Choreographing Engaged Encounters with Self and Other

In Move 3, the therapist uses the assembled, distilled, deepened emotion to set up engaged encounters with key others. Change involves a new experience and a new meaningful relationship event.

The therapist:

• Follows and accesses the emotional charge present in Move 2, distilling the client's new ordered emotion and noting how this emotion links to key dramas and the cast of characters that make up the existentially focused, identity-defining, present or past dramas in clients' lives. The emotional music sets up the dance of the new encounter.

• Sets up a new interactive, imaginal drama with an attachment figure or key part of self. The client is encouraged to vividly picture and engage with the other person (most often an attachment figure) or key part of self (often the most vulnerable or hurt part). The therapist develops this picture in detail so that clients can fully engage emotionally with this image.

• Encourages the client to share a clear statement of their core emotion with the imaginal figure or part of the self from these dramas. The therapist helps the client formulate the essence of their deeper emotion and state it with simple clarity and courage. Example: "Can you say to that small, scared, traumatized part of yourself hiding in the dark closet hardly daring to breathe, 'I see you and I feel so sad for you—I ache for you. You are so trapped. You are so afraid and so alone'." Or "Can you talk to your mother and hear her telling you, 'Don't feel. I don't want your soft, weak feelings—they are unacceptable.' The message that you heard is that if you feel, you will be rejected and you will hurt forever. Can you tell her, 'How could you leave me so alone and afraid? Act like I was nothing. This still hurts so much—I still long for your love, but it never appears'."

• Develops an absorbing core corrective emotional experience, deepening this new drama by constantly reflecting the client's key statements and asking simple questions to encourage the client to engage more fully. The therapist blocks exits and keeps the intensity of the drama going, all the while making sure to check with the client about their ability to tolerate or process this experience and when they need to be helped to bring closure and rest.

• Validates and normalizes clients' responses, summarizing the new experience that has emerged and distilling any new sense of self or capacity that has been discovered. The clinician especially notes how in previous interactional dramas, the client's self was negatively defined and a constrained emotional repertoire created, celebrating how the client is making changes and showing courage and competence. These changes are summarized and framed as key corrective experiences.

• Validates blocks that may emerge and any reluctance to engage with vulnerable core experience once it is evoked. The therapist helps the client own the difficulty and tell the key imagined other or part of self about it. The therapist could state something like, "You might say to her, 'This is too hard. I can't even let myself see your face or imagine telling you how small and scared I feel with you. It's too much'." The therapist accepts that for very good reasons the client is blocking at present, trusting that this acceptance will help the client engage at a later time. Clinical experience shows us that accepting and validating blocks tends to dissolve them.

- Searches for *positive resource moments* in a client's life where the client found a safe haven with another, or created an affirming, hope-generating experience in the face of overwhelming vulnerability. The therapist asks, "Was there ever a time of safety and comfort for you—someone who gave you a sense of hope?" or "Were there/are there any moments when you find a way to feel stronger and more confident?"

- Evokes and takes the client into this positive experience until it is vivid, asking the client to close their eyes and imagine it in detail so it can be felt.

- Summarizes and validates this positive experience and its survival consequences—impact on the sense of self, safety with others, and resilience. This is framed as a resource that the client can turn to as a safe haven and a secure base if and when the client feels overwhelmed. The therapist often returns to this and briefly evokes it in future sessions. Example: "Can you see your loving grandmother's face and hear her voice? What does she say to you? Can you take that in? She is telling you. . . . She helped you walk through that dark place and survive, and she is still here."

Early in therapy, Move 3 can be relatively superficial or light in nature, as when the therapist says, "Can you imagine saying this to your mum if she was here, Candice? Maybe just pause and imagine what that would feel like." Candice laughingly replies, "Oh no, I could never do that. I would be so terrified. I never express irritation or upset to her. I'd tell her, 'You are right mum,' and maybe she is." The therapist then gets Candice to just close her eyes for a moment and imagine saying to her mum, "You are always right, about me and about what I should feel and do." This deepens exploration and accustoms the client to this kind of intervention. However, as therapy continues, Move 3 becomes a potent, transformative, corrective emotional experience where new emotional realities are owned and enacted in significant contexts where the trauma unfolded, and the client's self and key emotional regulation strategies were defined. Saul tells me, "This feels like a dream. Telling my older brother that I am different, not him, but NOT weak or less than—not defective. I have carried this weight for two decades. Trying to protest and rage, then going into trying to please and hating myself for both. This is different. To speak my pain to him and to say who I am. It's bold. I feel stronger." Saul asserts who he is and the nature and validity of his experience to the one who, more than anyone else, he took as a model of manhood and arbiter of his worth. This is empowering at a deep emotional level. It signifies a new connection with self and a new positive way of enacting his emotions.

We must note that there are times, especially when working with life and death trauma, when the imagined other may be some version of Mother Nature, a spiritual or religious figure, a mentor, or some other representation of a key attachment. The therapist must be open to learning about the client and their particular culture and values, in order to be attuned and respectful to the client.

Move 4—Processing Encounters (New Identity Dramas)

In Move 4, the therapist focuses on and draws attention to the key aspects of change in the encounter. This is key always, but especially important in early phases of therapy when clients' views of self and other are likely to be entrenched, making any shifts difficult to recognize and own.

The therapist:

• Recounts the way clients assembled their emotional reality before Move 3 encounters in terms of their sense of self, relationships, and view of life, validating this reality as reasonable and valid in terms of the client's past experience.

Example: "How do you feel as we paint this picture—the spinning wheel of your emotions and how you had to deal with them up to now—the wheel that you have been caught on—stuck in, until today that is? It's natural that these new feelings and this new dance, way of being with yourself [or another if this is what occurred in Move 3] will seem strange to you." The wheel and patterned ways of relating are always framed as the problem, the trauma trap the client is caught in; the problem is not the client.

The client reflects on the process of Move 3, beginning to integrate it or reject it. "Yes—this is it. I got it. This is what I have done, how I have seen myself for the last 20 years. It helps to get this. Maybe I can dance a different dance now. What we did today feels totally different." Or "Yes but what is the point anyway? This is me and I will never change. Just talking about it will only make it worse."

• Summarizes, if integration is occurring, as vividly as possible and using the client's words, the new ways that the client organized their experience in the new drama that evolved in Move 3 of the Tango. The therapist asks the client to reflect on this and once again, feel into this.

• Validates and repeats the outline of the new script in the corrective drama and the new behavioral repertoire it offers. The therapist celebrates integration—the client's courage to open up to something new and to a new sense of who they are. The therapist also considers how difficult it is to absorb a new experience. Change and the uncertainty it brings is always scary.

• Validates blocks and explores them, if integration is problematic. Listing the fear of feeling new things and validating our common fears is often helpful. These may be formulated as: "Change is hard since it is walking from the familiar into the unknown"; "We fear that if we begin to feel, then we may be caught in hurt forever"; "Pain may then become ubiquitous and unbearable"; or "We may slip into chaos and craziness." It often just feels safer to stay with what you know. The therapist recognizes that the change process can be slow and involve only small steps toward the client's goals or can move quickly in a series of epiphanies. It is necessary to be always aware of the balance between safety and challenge and the need to titrate risk. One way to do this is simply to ask the client whether they were set too hard a task in Move 3 and learn from the feedback. As stated previously, the common clinical experience in EFT is that when blocks are accepted, explored, and validated, they begin to dissolve. To simply help the client return to Move 3 and acknowledge the block, telling the imagined other, "I just can't look at you or believe it's possible to say this to you," seems to be liberating.

In Move 4, the therapist is a witness to a new set of responses and plays them back to the client in a validating manner. This parallels what secure parents do naturally with a child who has risked a new set of responses. A mother might say, "Look what you did, Sammy. That is amazing! You were so brave." This process continues in Move 5.

Move 5—Integrate and Validate

In Move 5, the therapist draws attention to shifts in patterns as a means of highlighting and consolidating gains in session, as well as therapeutic gains over the course of therapy.

The therapist:

• Reflects and distills the client's progress in Moves 1 to 4 of the EFIT Tango, linking them to the client's problems and pain and integrating them into a positive picture of discovery and growth. The client has already made key changes by going through these moves. Their bravery and openness are celebrated; the reasonableness of their becoming caught in negative patterns of emotional and interpersonal patterns have been outlined. Their common shared humanity and vulnerability is honored. Growth is their birthright—they will be able to continue to evolve on this journey.

Throughout all the Moves of the Tango the iatrogenic traumatizing impact of emotional isolation, of rejection and abandonment, and of injuries by those who can hurt us the most is explicitly outlined and validated.

• Stresses that change is not in the future—it is already happening; the client is already changing. The therapist helps the client to explore the before and after of this process and formulate new responses in terms of positive self-esteem and compassion. As therapy evolves and changes become more significant, the therapist explores with the client what closure would look like in their EFIT process and if there are other issues that have not been addressed. The clinician also explores issues around relapse and what progress after therapy would look like. Short relapses are normalized and expected. However, the research on the EFT model suggests that changes hold years into the future. Once clients have tasted secure connection with self and others, they tend to hold onto it. The new resources they discover in therapy sessions foster a new relationship to the trauma story and cues that have structured their life up to this point.

Henny tells her therapist in their last sessions, "I don't go off somewhere else in my head now. I can stay if things get rough. I know when I am triggered and I know I can deal with it. My ex came round last night and started his usual diatribe about how I was just a traumatized, crazy fruit cake who no one could love, and this time, I just stood there and told him calmly, 'You never did understand my struggle but that is okay now. I know who I am and what happened to me, and I am fine. Now I want you to leave.' I felt like Superwoman." For a moment the therapist also feels the elation that Superwoman must feel when she makes the earth move.

<hr>

PLAY AND PRACTICE

For You Personally

Step 1

See if you can identify a traumatic moment in your life, perhaps a scary medical diagnosis or a car accident or any moment when, suddenly, you felt your whole life as you knew it was held in the balance. You can, of course, choose a more or less intense incident and engage more or less deeply here, whatever is best for you.

As you sit quietly and breathe in and out a few times to help you focus, can you identify the specific *trigger* (even in a long talk about a diagnosis there is often a word or phrase that our amygdala holds onto that feels like an electrifying alarm call), the immediate *perception* (e.g., falling or danger), the *body sensation,* the *cognitions,* what you said to yourself (often catastrophizing), and the impulse or *action tendency* that emerged, what you wanted to do?

Breathing softly again for a few breaths, can you listen to this music and put your finger on a word that captures the deepest emotional response that you are aware of right now? For example, Jenny described her response when told she had a very dangerous form of cancer as "dumbstruck, helpless, pinned to the wall."

What did you do to cope with these feelings at the time?

How do you cope with these feelings now? What impact does your way of dealing with these emotions have on your life?

Step 2

Often, even when we can feel into, accept, and specify our most difficult vulnerable feelings, it is hard to speak of them to another, to make them explicit and own them.

Try to pinpoint and coherently and succinctly share your felt experience with a key person in your life. What happened to you, your feelings, your body, your sense of self as you did this? If this sharing was too hard to do, can you see yourself telling this person or figure what made it too hard to do?

How did this person respond to you? Were they open and responsive or . . . ?

If your response to the above was, "No, I have never shared my truest emotion about this traumatic moment," then can you access what keeps you from sharing this? What is the worst thing that could happen if you share?

Finally, what has it been like to do this exercise? What have you learned?

For You Professionally

How would you pinpoint the core essential emotion in the following remarks made by Susie? What would you say?

SUSIE: I get triggered every time. I cannot help it! Any hint of criticism sends me into the same spiral I fell in when I was 4 years old and learning to play the piano. I end up lashing out, then feeling guilty, alone, and misunderstood again and again. What's the point? I feel like I should just give up. I will never be the friend, partner, parent I would like to be.

The therapist now highlights trigger and response. What would you say, and how would you next intervene?

SUSIE: Yes, that's it. (*Tears now start to well in her eyes.*)

The therapist now moves toward deepening. What would you do? What would you say?

How would you summarize this poignantly into a clear, focused message to a safe other? How would you summarize this message if it was directed to the most vulnerable part of self by a stronger more confident and resourced part of self?

Describe a positive outcome for this encounter and its impact on the client.

KEY TAKEAWAYS

Three Threads Are Integrated into the Tapestry That Is a Therapy Session

1. Attachment science and the map to human function it provides.
2. The interventions outlined by Carl Rogers who believed, like Bowlby, that empathic relationships are healing, and provide the resilience and growth that are our birthright.
3. Clinical knowledge gained from 35 years of practice and research on EFT as an effective model of intervention.

The EFT Tango

The EFT Tango is:

- a dance of attunement;
- a set of macro interventions used, often repeatedly, throughout the three stages of therapy;
- implemented at varying levels of intensity across therapy stages and sessions; and
- a metaphor that captures an alive, moving process of growth.

The EFT Tango is NOT:

■ a mechanical set of interventions to be done in sequence;
■ used in a specific sequence at the same level of depth across stages of therapy; and
■ static and one-dimensional.

The EFT Tango Has Five Moves

Move 1: Reflecting Present Process
Move 2: Assembling and Deepening Emotion
Move 3: Choreographing Engaged Encounters
Move 4: Processing the Encounter
Move 5: Integrating and Validating

Preparation for the Tango

Send attuned safe-haven signals.
Tune into key moments/pivotal experiences that have shaped attachment.
Reflect both suffering and coping strategies.
Unpack abstract symptom labels and find the logic in symptoms and difficulties.
Gauge client capacity, reach for competence, and set up expectations for success.
Be transparent and collaborative.

Choreographing the Encounter with FACES

Frame and focus. Create a context.
Anticipate contact and the desired outcome.
Care and safety—create and maintain.
Engage the encounter—make the request/invite or guide the client.
Stay the course. Make space for deepening. Address blocks. Attend to window of tolerance/capacity.

4

Key EFT Assumptions
and Micro Interventions

It is useful to remember that when a path is laid out for us by past experiences of safe connection with self and others, we are more resilient. That means that coping and change can unfold naturally in the face of trauma and severe stress. When we have grown in the context of secure connection, as troubles come up, we find a place to stand with a trusted other who holds and grounds us with their presence. We begin to see how our hearts and minds can spin into recurring patterns and protocols, and how these patterns can become expectations and stories that run our lives and run us into the ground. We can focus our attention and identify and taste the deeper emotions, like fear and sadness, that shape our stories, and we can accept their logic. We then can bring these emotions to life in our interactions with the most vulnerable parts of ourselves and with special others, making them more concrete and real, and expanding our sense of self. When we operate from a place of safety, we can reflect on this whole process and take it in, trusting in it and in ourselves. This is what the more securely connected of us seem to be able to do naturally in times of turmoil and stress in order to reach for resilience. The writings on the practice of mindfulness touch on this natural process of change, where experience is engaged with in an open, accepting way, and an awareness of how it is being constructed by the experiencer is made clear so that new levels of experience can emerge (e.g., see Kabat-Zinn, 2003, 2024; Rosenbaum & Bohart, 2021). These new levels of awareness lead to acceptance and self-compassion and strengthen our ability to handle suffering.

Even though this process of finding our way through overwhelming events to a new integration may unfold naturally, at times it is not easy and many of us need a guide—a therapist—to help us see and walk this path. This is not an admission of any kind of weakness or lack of character, rather, it is an honoring of our natural desire to avoid meeting monsters alone and to find a secure base to help us grow.

What we have just described in simple terms is the exact process of positive change in EFT and EFIT in particular. However, for a health professional to guide someone through this process, we need to look at it in detail. We first offer a general snapshot of the assumptions and core practice principles of EFIT and then turn to describing specific interventions.

EIGHT BASIC ASSUMPTIONS
FOR HEALING THE WOUNDS OF TRAUMA

The following eight assumptions, taken from the attachment perspective, the humanistic framework of Carl Rogers, and the practice of the EFT model, are essential to structure a healing framework for the wounds of trauma.

1. *All clients are capable of growth and increased resilience if offered a safe, validating context where their stuck places and dead-end dilemmas are recognized, accepted, and explored.* Safety for the trauma client is especially crucial since many have absolutely no reason to trust another and are exceptionally wary of engagement with their own inner world since that is where their inner demons reside. In EFIT, the client is continually framed as worthy and competent.

It behooves the therapist to constantly attend to pacing and to a client's window of tolerance, gauging the working distance from difficult emotional experience, the distance between what is tolerable and intolerable. The therapist tells Yan, "This is so hard. Let's go really slow here and you can tell me if it is too much. I am feeling with you now. You must always tell me if our work here becomes too hard for you. You can tell me, 'I don't want to touch this,' that is fine. You are so brave to even begin to move closer to this nightmare. But you are doing it, right here."

2. *The goal of therapy is more than symptom management, it is an increased sense of balance and groundedness, which then fosters a secure sense of connection with self and others.* This is captured in Roger's concept of existential living, where there is an openness and ability to manage experience so that life is vibrant, tangible, and full.

So, the therapist tells Saul, "Yes, I understand that this is where you live, in all this chaos. It makes sense. No one ever stood with you and helped you grasp what was happening. But right now, you are with me, and we are naming these sensations and images and thoughts as 'panic,' and you are gradually opening the door to it with courage. It is specific isn't it, clear? This is what you felt in those moments when your father picked up his belt, or now when your partner scrunches her face in anger. You are naming this and touching it here with me and making it clear. And as you gain this awareness, you can more readily regain your balance in moments of distress."

3. *The therapy relationship must be genuine, transparent, empathically responsive, and collaborative. It must be an ARE relationship where the therapist is accessible, responsive, and genuinely engaged with the client as a caring other.* The essence of effective therapeutic interaction is sensitive attunement. To achieve this, the therapist has to be genuinely curious and willing to explore and feel the struggles of each particular client as an individual, not as an example of a group labeled with an abstract disorder. The therapist follows the client and leads, creating the dance of the session, asking for the client's help in understanding their pain and willingness to engage in the process of the session.

The therapist might say, "Help me understand. This is the point where you 'numb out' so you cannot even see in your mind's eye the faces of the people in this scene. It is all 'foggy.' This is the point in your story where your body screams danger and the only way to survive is to shut down, to go away. Is this right? What is it like for you to hear me say this? Can you hear me? We can stop here right now if you wish. Your face looks a little tight. Is this maybe too scary or is it about stopping sad tears, maybe, or?"

In this same vein, the therapist is willing to be transparent, explaining, for example, why they are asking the client to focus on a particular topic or close their eyes to engage more deeply with an emotional image or moment. As well, when the client expresses hesitation or uncertainty, transparency offers choice—agency—in and of itself a corrective emotional experience.

4. *Emotion is not seen as a problem per se—the therapist befriends it. It is not simply commented on or bypassed but is honored, tracked, and held up to the light with repeated empathic reflections so that it becomes less frightening, less alien, and less unacceptable.* It is focused on and evoked but is also regulated by the therapist's manner and presence. For the therapist and client, emotion provides a compass that outlines distressing stuck places and indicates new responses that lead forward. When lost in a session, the therapist can regain focus by going back to the last word or emotional response that resonated with the

client, moving the client into the deeper more core emotions that organize their world. Trauma cues become clear, as does their existential significance. As stated previously, the awareness of new or more elaborated emotions also cues new action tendencies, such as grieving for or comforting the self or assertively protesting against traumatic abuse by others. This awareness also helps clients recognize and deal with both their vulnerabilities and their needs.

The therapist says, "Right. These reflections on your moments of irritation are important but can we just go back a moment? You said you feel burned, your face changed, and then you teared up. Burned. Can we stay here for a moment? Burns hurt and they scare us—sear us. They are dangerous. As you say this, what happens?"

The client responds, "I can't breathe. I see my father yelling at me and saying, 'Look what you did! Don't upset your mother, you selfish, disgusting little brat. She is fragile.' He doesn't see me at all. It scalds me. That is the story of my childhood." This client, who presented with an anger problem, now weeps and accesses the isolation and longings of their more vulnerable self, emotions that they usually keep hidden even from themself. As they do this, they change the level of their engagement with their emotions and their relationship to them; previously denied and fragmented feelings are accessed and tolerated. The client can then follow these emotions into the pain of their childhood loneliness and deprivation. This becomes a compass pointing to the possibility of embracing their denigrated traumatized self and cueing self-compassion, rather than their habitual self-disgust.

5. *The PROCESS of moving from key blocks into development and growth unfolds in each session. The therapist has to track content and process—the how of things.* The therapist finds and specifies the PATTERNS of recurring inner emotional responses and ineffectual attempts at regulation that simply keep the client on an ever-turning wheel of distress—a self-sustaining feedback loop of attempted protection from distress that leads nowhere. Interpersonal patterns of engagement with others also merge with and reinforce these emotional patterns. It is these patterns that keep the client from moving forward into posttraumatic growth. Again, the therapist looks for the organizing elements, or steps, in the dance with self and others, rather than just outlining content. These patterns are the context where the self is defined as helpless and unworthy. It is empowering for the client to grasp the structure of their inner and relational world, that is, to see HOW they are constructing their ongoing experience and relationships in a way that constricts them. This awareness can shift the pattern, but it also changes the client's relationship to the pattern. As Amy says to her therapist, "I

get that this is a dance that just repeats itself, that I am caught in. It is not *me*." Such emotional and relational patterns have to be normalized in therapy. They are, as Bowlby reminds us, "perfectly rational" given the context in which they arose. We all have such habitual blueprints, but trauma elicits such compelling cues and responses that awareness and flexibility are almost always out of reach. The PRESENCE of the therapist aids in the focus on PRESENT MOMENT, the PRIMARY/ CORE AFFECT, the PROCESS, and PATTERNS in a *nonpathologizing* manner. These are often referred to as the 5 P's of EFIT and EFT. Identifying these patterns helps us make sense of the client's inability to move beyond trauma without pathologizing.

The therapist says at the end of the first session, "So Pam, if I am hearing correctly, you are caught in a dance of being triggered by any sign of rejection or anger from others, and at the first hint of this, you simply shut down. It seems there is nothing else to do. You go into 'paralysis,' is what you said. As you do this, you seem distant and so others move away from you, confirming your worst fears. Then you go home and space out on dope and food and video games. Have I got it? But this brings waves of self-doubt and self-disgust, so you are more and more sensitive and want to hide even more." The client then refines this formulation, and the therapist uses this refined version again and again in session.

6. *The therapist recognizes that, just as emotional connection with safe others protects against feelings of helplessness and meaninglessness, isolation renders us much more vulnerable and feeds these responses; responses that are key features of PTSD.* Isolation is then particularly noted and its impact is explored with clients. This is a way into normalizing trauma responses and their impact, and cueing clients into their deprivation and longing for contact. Recognizing this longing motivates self-compassion, growth, and risk taking.

The therapist says, "Of course your body says 'run' when we approach this topic, Alexa. We are not wired to face such dragons alone and you were always alone, weren't you? You were never seen or held or protected. You never had any alternative but to 'smother yourself' as you say. We are so much more vulnerable when we sense that there is no one who will come when we call. I feel it in my chest when you talk about holding your dog and rocking. That was the only comfort you had. So of course, you could not do what you tell yourself you should have done, which is to fight and rage and assert yourself. And now you long for closeness but it's hard to trust and to let people in—yes? It is terrifying to feel so alone."

An acknowledgment of the power of our need for others and the devastation of emotional isolation helps a therapist understand the import of what we have called *attachment injuries,* which are relational traumas. These are abandonments or rejections at key moments of need by the attachment figures to whom we turn for comfort and reassurance. They deliver the message that the abandoned person does not matter, is not valued, and cannot expect support from others in times of greatest vulnerability. So, a wife may forgive a brief affair but not forgive her partner's choice to lead a sports team in a big final that resulted in her giving birth to her first child without her partner's support. A trauma survivor may find a way to compartmentalize her rape at the hands of her drunken father, but it is the image of her mother calmly walking out of the room rather than coming to her aid that tortures her.

7. *Trauma clients often reach a point where they are simply depleted, exhausted, and constantly overwhelmed. The competent therapist must do what loving attachment figures do: They constantly validate and systematically act as a resource to the suffering survivor.* This support is an antidote to the shame and self-blame that accompanies so much trauma, but it also creates hope and models compassionate responses to the client. The concept of resourcing the client can be viewed in attachment terms as the finding and expanding awareness of moments of comfort and safety in the past or present in the client's life that they can turn to when distressed in session and at home. Moments of risk and competence can also be discovered, and the experience accessed and tuned into in session so it is alive and can be used to calm and protect the client. This validation and resource provision not only help regulate difficult emotions, they also offer the client a new positive image of themselves that empowers them.

The therapist says, "I understand. Of course, you berate yourself and tell yourself you are unacceptable and deficient—this was the constant message you received from those you depended on. And of course, you cannot 'see' how much you were hurt and how you are worth crying for—no one saw you, did they, and no one heard your pain and made it matter. But you survived and you are here working on this. You look at your difficulties here with me and you are honest and struggling to grow. Can we go back to those moments of safety with your grandmother that you remembered in the last session? She called you, 'Special Magic One—Princess,' and you remember her voice, soft and warm and her arms around you. Can you close your eyes and feel that now? Yes. This is a safe place to come home to, isn't it? She saw you and you mattered to her. She was proud of you. You remembered her when you were scared to sign the form to attend college, and you stepped out of your fear and signed it. She helped you find your courage."

8. *Corrective emotional experiences foster growth and take the client past the dead-ends of trauma. Deep emotional engagement and exploration and the epiphanies it brings are the primary engine of lasting change.* In such transformative moments, vulnerability is encountered with balance and confidence. A coherent sense of a competent worthy self emerges and begins to be consolidated. Patterns of engagement that make up the relationship with self and with others shift in a positive direction. Here, it helps tremendously if the guiding other (a loving attachment figure or a surrogate attachment figure such as a therapist) understands the way such moments of intense transformation are structured. In such transforming moments, core vulnerabilities are experienced fully and coherently expressed, and the accompanying needs accepted and asserted. Key elements of traumatic experience come online and are changed by the addition of new emotions, insights, and action tendencies. This experience is best played out as a vivid drama with elements of self or important others whose messages constantly whisper in our ear and play a key part in how we define ourselves. As EFIT therapists and researchers observe such events, it has become clearer and clearer, as is consonant with attachment science, that they constitute *identity dialogues* and help shift the client's model of self in a positive direction. This process happens naturally in secure attachment relationships but can also be structured in therapy sessions. They offer a predictable way through the darkness and a sense of completion as regards to traumatic events, communicating to the client that life can begin anew.

The therapist says to Sarah, "So you wake in the night struggling with all this self doubt, with all this judgment echoing in your ears and telling you not to take this new job and not to trust this new man. The voice says you are 'bad, destructive, and do not deserve things like this.' But now you don't just shut down, you know what is happening and you know the pain that is behind all this. Can you feel this struggle now— how your body tenses and strains? Do you know whose voice it is you hear? (*Client nods.*) Good."

The client weeps and reiterates images of the hurt, frailty, and helplessness that come along with this voice and how she has concurred with its judgments for years while denying her own hurts and needs. She articulates the most painful message of all, the one that sends her "over the cliff" and finds, to her surprise, that it is not her religious father's voice but that of her older sister publicly listing her sins and shortcomings after what was deemed an inappropriate display of sexuality. As this voice becomes clear, she is able to steady herself, respond to and legitimize her own pain, and find a coherent assertive response that she gradually puts together and turns into an imagined drama with her sister. As this plays out, she finds that she now deems herself as worthy, not just of "forgiveness" but of respect and love, and she asserts this. The therapist helps her integrate and consolidate this experience and validates her struggle and her new discoveries. After the session ends, she is able to risk reaching for loving connection in her life, suddenly sure of who she is and that she is entitled to respect and caring after all.

EXPERIENTIAL THERAPIST SKILLS
AND MICRO INTERVENTIONS IN EFT

Most therapies and natural recovery processes after trauma seem to proceed through three basic stages (Herman, 1992): the attainment and maintenance of some measure of balance and ability to look at and explore difficult experience, which can be titled *Stabilization;* the *Restructuring* of the trauma experience; and the *Consolidation* of change and recovery. EFIT also evolves in these three stages. By the end of Stabilization (Stage 1), clients show less of what Barlow notes as the core features of all emotional disorders (Barlow et al., 2004; Barlow, 2011), that is, they show less tendency to be hijacked by chaotic negative emotion, less avoidance of any reminders of vulnerability or trauma, less vigilance for threat, and less negativity about the self. In Restructuring (Stage 2), they develop more ability to tune into their inner and relational experience, acquire more openness to deeply engage in exploration at the edge of that experience, and show more willingness to take risks and move into what is frightening, alien, and unacceptable. By Consolidation (Stage 3), they demonstrate more trust in themselves as being strong enough to cope with pain and fear and are less caught in negative identity traps. They develop a stronger more secure connection to themselves and others.

No matter what the stage of therapy, there are certain general skills and ways of responding that are used in EFT that are especially pertinent when treating the intense vulnerability associated with trauma (Johnson & Campbell, 2022). These behaviors often show up in positive attachment relationships in general, but the therapist uses them more predictably, consciously, and deliberately. In EFIT, the main source of these skilled practices, apart from over three decades of clinical practice, is the work of Carl Rogers. Therapists use these practices to make primary core experience more accessible, specific, concrete, tangible, manageable, and acceptable; that is, to lead the client into an awareness of how experience is constructed and either opens out into continual learning and growth or narrows down into constriction and dysfunction.

Interventions are used in such a way as to follow the Buddhist principle that "the only way out is through" and to create what the Buddha called "the sure heart's release" (Goldstein, 1993).

Reflection—Empathic and On Target

The main practice skill that Rogers and the EFT model are known for is so simple that it is often discounted or even mocked. It is the continuous *reflection* of a client's ongoing experience as it is being encoded, felt, and expressed in the present moment. Bowlby also spoke of inner, emotionally loaded experience as a "felt sense," that is, as an embodied alive event, not as simply a set of cognitions or as information processing. Rogers (1961) famously stated that "a good reflection is not a repetition, but a revelation."

Over three decades of therapy and many outcome and process of change research studies have persuaded us that Rogers was right. The EFIT therapist constantly tunes into the client's experience as expressed, both the verbal and nonverbal cues, and feeds them back to the client (as in Rogers amplified). The therapist sifts through what they hear and focuses on the signals that are pertinent to the client's emotional state, reported symptoms or distress, relationships with others, and identity. This reflecting is done respectfully and in a way that is open to correction. Done well, it holds up a mirror, giving a clear, organized view of the client's experience.

Reflection is revelatory in that it continually focuses clients on the key elements of what is happening and on how they encode events and meaning. The therapist may simply listen to many stories and comments about content issues but then repeat, focus on, and return to the one poignant emotional phrase used by the client that is common in all the issues. Tara tells her therapist about her siblings and the details of her job, her diagnoses, and her husband's job from a detached, information-giving stance. But then she laughs and slips in, "I don't know what is wrong with me. Nothing makes sense. I am useless—not of value." The EFIT therapist will slow down, lean in, and repeat this remark, often going on to ask a simple question. This is especially crucial with trauma clients since they often offer rambling tangential narratives and avoid the painful organizing center of their story. For example, Saul tells his therapist, "I know I am difficult. I go off in ten directions at once and I add and qualify stuff, and I interrupt you. No one can handle me. But you seem to be able to stay focused on what matters and that helps. I get the feeling we are going somewhere. How do you do that?" The answer is simple but profound. Reflection slows down the conversation and allows the therapist to taste and order the client's experience, giving time to consider a response, and helping the therapist move past any irritation at a continually tangential client!

Empathic reflections continually organize and order a client's experience so that this experience is more manageable and can be seen more clearly. The therapist highlights the main themes in the client's chaotic narratives at the beginning of therapy, pointing out self-reinforcing patterns that shape pain and distress. Throughout therapy, repetitive reflection also soothes the nervous system and helps it orient to and take in a message. We see this with lullabies, in poetry, in song lyrics, and in prayer and rituals. In EFT, we are trying to sing to the lower parts of the brain. We know that the brain on high alert does not hear the first reflection, dismisses the second, hears the next one as less threatening and starts to let it in, and then upon hearing the fourth or fifth reflection, resonates with the message and considers its impact and meaning. In short, reflections are most powerful when used with quiet persistence.

On the most basic level, empathic reflections create safety. They build and maintain a therapeutic alliance. The meta-messages inherent in accurate, attuned reflections are extremely supportive and even seductive. They implicitly communicate, "I see you. I am here. Your message matters to me. I can sort out and respond to what matters most. You are not alone with this. You are safe with me." Being able to confront trauma depends on this safety.

Reflections also build emotional momentum while ordering the flow of experience and at the same time, holding the client in a safe place. Constantly returning to key phrases the client has used, what we call *emotional handles* in EFT, keeps clients focused on the path into and through their pain. It prevents both client and therapist from getting lost in details or irrelevancies, and it builds intensity. It also sets the stage for the corrective emotional epiphanies that are at the heart of change in EFIT.

Blocks and exits from engagement in the therapy process are also reflected and the logic of such self-protective moves is validated. Ironically, this nearly always fosters a willingness to risk and begin to follow the therapist's lead into difficult territory. The therapist might comment, "I notice that when we get to this point and your sadness comes up, Jean, that you move into tidying your desk and bringing in another topic. You have said that you are not sure you want to get any closer to these feelings. That is very natural. It is so hard to open up to such hurt and you have never felt safe enough to do that—yes? We can talk about how hard this is and what you tell yourself might happen if we do walk slowly into this place."

In short, repeated empathic reflection is the simplest, and by far the most useful, tool for keeping focus and directing progress that we have ever found in psychotherapy. It is fascinating how young therapists sometimes tell us that it feels awkward or superfluous. Perhaps the key issue is that if you are on target, then repetition deepens experience and engagement, inviting clients into the flow of deep emotions and their personal, defining dramas. As a therapist, to be confident that you are on target, you need a map to the structure of emotions, relationship interactions and their effects, human needs, and the process of development and change, addressed earlier and which will continue to be addressed in this text.

Evocative Questions

The therapist begins by meeting clients where they are in the present. Very often this means meeting them in general discussion or listening to surface reactive emotions. However, it is not long before a competent therapist begins to expand and deepen the emotional music behind the client's main symptoms and relational dance moves, eliciting underlying emotions, thoughts and motivations, and outlining the ways in which clients are constructing their experience. The easiest way to do this is to ask simple, evocative, process-oriented questions, such as *what, when,* and *how.* These process-oriented enquiries literally invite or evoke experiential exploration, especially into immediate experiencing, emotions, and the client's history of threat/danger and safety. In the beginning, they can be relatively content-oriented, as in, "Who did you feel safe with or go to for comfort as a child?" But then expand into exploring concrete experience with a question like, "How do you reassure or comfort yourself now?" Such questions tune into a wealth of information relevant to emotion regulation, trauma symptoms, relationship patterns, and models of self. As therapy continues, these questions are often present-oriented, as in, "How do you feel as we talk about this or as I ask you to stay with this topic?" or "What do you say to yourself when these triggers flood you and you feel this burn across your chest?" In EFIT, the question *why* is avoided since it elicits top-down abstract cognitive perspectives.

Validation

This affirmation of the client's difficulties, stuck patterns, present efforts and strengths shown in session or in their life story, provides a sense of safety and an ongoing antidote to the impacts of trauma. This validation provides more than encouragement and hope; it also offers an alternative way of viewing reality. Specifically, it normalizes and places the client's struggles in the context of the deprivation of attachment needs and longings, the pain of isolation, and a lack of belonging. The script, "I must be at fault and uniquely defective and undeserving," can then be softened and expanded into, "We are all vulnerable and all find ourselves caught, at times, in a terrible helplessness and lack of options in our lives. We are all afraid of failing with others or finding ourselves invisible and of no consequence."

The tenor of this validation is not the same as praise, and it is not the traditional formal positive feedback offered by a teacher. Rather, it is more in line with how a supportive, engaged mother talks to an unsure and hesitant child who is taking a risk or even the way we seem to sometimes enthusiastically talk to our dogs! It is personal, generous, and sincere, validating any difficulty and expressing delight in any step forward or even in the ability to tolerate risk and survive. A therapist might say to a client, "You are so courageous, Aya. I understand how hard this is for you and that you need to go very slow here—stop short of really picturing yourself as a terrified little one, avert your eyes from seeing this little girl's face. That little one, she was so alone, wasn't she, and she felt so helpless—had no safe place at all. It is good to protect yourself, to make sure you want to do this. I know you are strong enough to do it but it's good to take it slow." The desire to protect oneself and block the risks unfolding in a particular therapy session are also validated and the logic of this desire accepted. The therapist empathically accepts the client's blocks to emotional engagement in session and finds the logic in the client's response.

Interpretation

An empathic listener who tunes into another's experience often naturally adds a conjecture, expanding the picture of this experience to help make the experience whole or more meaningful. So a therapist might tentatively suggest a clearer emotional response, as in, "It sounds like, as you said, this experience became a little too much. Maybe even a little scary, overwhelming?" If the therapist wants to increase intensity or make the implicit more explicit, this small addition at the leading edge of a client's experience can be stated in proxy voice, that is, as if the client is the one who is speaking; for example, "I hear you saying, 'Oh this is confusing.' And perhaps, it's almost like those other times when there is a voice in your head saying, 'I am so unsure here. I am going to mess this up and then I will know that I am not enough—that I am just a failure'?"

Good interpretations stay close to the client's experience. They are not abstract intellectual comments and do not add too much to a client's remarks so as not to wander into territory that is alien or that the client is not open to considering. Often a client will take in the therapist's addition to the description of their experience but then correct it, making it more personal or exact. The therapist might say, "I hear that in these difficult incidents and conflicts, you tell yourself that you have somehow let everyone down?" The client replies, "Let them down—oh, more than that. I am a despicable traitor." The conjecture expands the frame and invites the client to deepen their awareness and ability to capture their experience. In a collaborative therapy, it is also possible to ask for help in understanding a client's experience and in the process, offer some connecting conjectures for the client's consideration. The therapist might say, "Can you help me here? It almost sounds like when you lose your cool with your lady, it is like your description of your experience as a child. You said that you so wanted to please but there was also the feeling of being taken over or smothered by having to take care of someone else's need, no matter how you felt? So naturally you want to protest and push the person away. Is this it or . . . maybe I am not understanding?"

Deepening Engagement in a Moment or an Emotion

These techniques are used especially in Move 2 of the EFIT Tango, Affect Assembly, and Deepening, to access core emotions and are particularly useful when preparing the client to segue into Move 3, where emotionally engaged clients move into and enact a corrective emotional drama. The therapist zeros in on a key moment or emotional response that is particularly significant and relevant to the client's dilemmas and distress. The goal is to encourage the client to stay with and actively feel and explore this moment. The ways to do this are simple but powerful when used with intention and persistence. It is crucial that these moves are enacted in an extremely supportive manner, preferably in a soft, slow voice and in simple, specific language. As mentioned previously, in EFT we call this "singing to the amygdala." As the client touches profound pain or fear, the emotional music the therapist plays is soothing and evokes the contact comfort associated with secure attachment interactions. We offer a summary of these micro interventions that facilitate deepening engagement, many of which have already been mentioned:

• Reflection and Repetition, often—of the client's words or emotional handles, perhaps with an interpretive edge given by the therapist. The therapist says, "Yes, you used the word 'trapped' again here. 'Trapped,' as you said before, 'in all that aloneness, suffering silently, helpless with no one to turn to, trying to hide and not be there—holding your doll under your bed. Trapped and alone.' That is so hard. Terrifying even." Here the word "terrifying" is a conjecture, an interpretation. The therapist routinely writes down a client's potent words that capture key trauma experiences, such as "trapped," and then uses them again and again as handles to open the door into deeper experience.

• Evocative questioning as outlined above, focused on present experience. The therapist says, "What is happening right now, Ellen, right now in your body as we talk about this?"

• The use of evocative imagery or metaphor to capture meaning and make it more poignant. The therapist uses their imagination as triggered by their own empathic attunement to the client's experience or expands on and makes more vivid an image already given by the client, perhaps in another session. The therapist comments, "I hear echoes of that image you offered a while ago from a dream you had. You are treading water out in the ocean, barely staying afloat. But your sisters are drowning around you, and you desperately swim to each of them to try to hold them up, hold them up so they can breathe. But you are all drowning, aren't you, in the sea of terror of your father's attacks, fighting for your life and trying to save your sisters at the same time. As I see this, a kind of desperation comes up in me but maybe that is just me?"

• The use of proxy voice—speaking as the client—intensifies experience. When the therapist accurately echoes a client's emerging emotional experience in the first person, this offers a direct, up close, coherent version of their inner experience that invites deeper engagement. It is best to do this only when the therapist has a clear, specific sense of a client's core emotions and their significance for process patterns and the manner in which clients define themselves. The use of a soft, slow voice and accurate empathy is essential here.

With trauma survivors in particular, it is necessary to keep each client's window of tolerance in mind when deepening/heightening engagement with distressing emotions or moments. Therapists take their cue from their client's responses and titrate the "dose" of intensity so that there is, what Gendlin (1996) called, a "working distance" from emotion. Pacing follows the client's ability to stay grounded and open to direction and soothing. Much like a safe attachment figure supports a child to confront a fear and take a risk but then is careful not to overwhelm the child, the therapist tunes into what the client can tolerate and use at any point in time. It is also possible to slice risks thinner if a client begins to be overwhelmed by simply exploring the nature of the risk itself. The EFIT therapist uses deepening carefully and attunes to a client's ability to engage and manage risk. Being aware of the seven different levels of experiencing also helps and are a part of the ongoing assessment process in EFIT.

Reframing

Cognitive reframes are part of EFIT and are usually used to normalize problematic responses or cycles or organize underlying emotion into a model of patterned responses. So, as Saul talks about himself as a "traitor" and "betrayer who disappointed his family," the therapist continually reflects his pain and frames him as deserving of compassion, since he was caught between being a strongman for his father and brother, and a comforting but dependent child figure for his mother—an impossible set of competing expectations. This reflection and reframe only works if the accompanying emotions are engaged and relevant. With Saul, this reframe fits and begins to interfere with and offer an alternative to his self-disgust because he is beginning to access his desperate longing to please and his fear of disappointing others. The new frame is guided by attachment science and the EFIT model.

Reflecting, Tracking, and Directly Choreographing Unfolding Dramas

Interactions with present and past attachment figures, with figures central to a client's trauma, and also with elements of self, are enacted in Move 3 of the EFIT Tango: Choreographing Engaged Encounters. This requires the therapist to play the part of collaborative choreographer, setting up the emotional music and directing the moves in an evolving dance as it glides toward an emotional epiphany. Therapists often ask how they can know what other figure or part of the client's self to choose when setting up this kind of drama. The answer is that the client will tell you. Following the client's process will lead the therapist to the part of self, internal figure, or present person in the client's life that has the most emotional significance. Also, if the therapist helps a client choose a focus and it does not evolve into an engaging drama, then the therapist can simply redirect, return to exploring affect, and choose another figure. These imaginal dramas often start out early in therapy with a short, rather superficial interaction with a less important person in the client's life, allowing the client to get used to the nature of these interventions. But this changes as therapy continues. In the most moving and relevant interactions, clients will access figures with whom they are swept into poignant new dramas where they voice their pain and longings and access new emotional responses. These are also the figures with whom they need to find a new way to communicate and relate in order to be able to redefine themselves. In EFIT with trauma clients, especially those suffering from complex PTSD and childhood maltreatment, most often the key transforming drama is enacted with the most vulnerable, helpless part of self and the now agentic and coherent adult self who is resourced by the therapist. These dramas constitute Move 3 of the EFIT Tango, as addressed in the previous chapter. Suffice to say that these dramas are longer and more intense in Stage 2 (Restructuring), than in Stage 1—(Stabilization), and that intensity also varies with each client and each client's style. The therapist needs a solid alliance, the ability to help the client engage openly with their deeper emotion, and a sense of how to keep focus and how to structure these dramas so that they develop into a corrective experience.

To reiterate, in all of the above interventions, it matters HOW they are presented. The music of a message, the tone, tenor, and pacing, decides how the information in the message is received and processed. As we've written elsewhere (Johnson & Campbell, 2022), "Clients will most often not take the risk of deepening their engagement with their vulnerabilities or hanging out at the leading edge of what is known to discover new territory if the therapist goes too fast, uses many abstract intellectual words, or speaks in an impersonal externally oriented tone of voice." The quality of the therapist's responses and voice is particularly relevant for survivors who need constant reassurance that they are safe and connected with an available, supportive other. A useful mantra here, especially with trauma clients, is Soft, Slow, Simple, and Specific. The best way to really know how a person comes across as a therapist is for this person to watch their own therapy videos. Both authors have practiced this over many years and learned immeasurably valuable lessons from this process, in particular, to slow down, to persevere, and to repeat interventions. Focus and momentum are the cornerstone of effective therapy of any type and with all clients.

PLAY AND PRACTICE

For You Personally

Our messages to loved ones often get lost when we speak in a hurried manner or with a tone of aggression or exasperation. Our words might be on target, but if they are not delivered with attention to pace and grace, they can often sabotage our intent and leave us feeling unseen and unheard, and ultimately, with our needs unmet. Think about a recent example of such an experience. You might have been on the receiving end of such scrambled messages or the communicator. What was the message that you were trying to convey or that you think your loved one was attempting to communicate? Can you identify the core emotion that was confused by surface emotion or other process elements? Are you able to identify the need that might have been met had the message been delivered differently? As comfortable, share this with your loved one as a form of repair or corrective emotional experience.

For You Professionally

Seek permission from a client to videotape a session. Review the tape with specific attention to process elements (your own and the client's) such as tone, facial expression, speech, affect. Write notes. What do you notice you could improve upon? Write out three goals for your next sessions.

KEY TAKEAWAYS

Eight Basic Assumptions for Healing the Wounds of Trauma

1. All clients are capable of growth and resilience if offered safety and security.
2. The goal of therapy is more than symptom management; it is a secure connection with self and others.
3. The therapy relationship must be genuine, transparent, empathically responsive, and collaborative. That is, the therapist must be ARE: Accessible, Responsive, and Engaged.
4. Emotion is prioritized.
5. The therapist tracks content and process.
6. The therapist acknowledges the power of our need for others and the devastation of emotional isolation, especially during times of need.
7. The therapist resources the client with self and others
8. Corrective emotional experiences foster growth.

The Five Ps in EFT

Presence of the therapist
Present Moment
Primary/Core Affect
Process
Patterns

Three Stages of EFT

Stabilization
Restructuring
Consolidation

Key Skills/EFT Micro Interventions

Reflection
Evocative Questions
Validation
Interpretation
Evocative imagery or metaphor to capture meaning
Use of proxy voice
Reframing

5

Assessment as a Guide through
the Three Stages of EFIT Intervention

Initial sessions with Sierra reveal enormous potential thwarted by a series of experiences that have colored her perceptions of self and the world as negative, shrunk her ability to tune into and trust her internal experience, and restricted her capacity to love and be loved. All signs of insecure attachment. Now in her late 30s, she is pursuing therapy at the urging of her wife, who is seeking a stronger emotional connection. Currently embracing yet another chance at life following liver failure and a transplant, Sierra is willing to attend an initial session or two but is not optimistic about therapy. Her prior experiences with mental health professionals of the dominant culture have been extensive but limiting, leading to an array of diagnoses, *trauma by some other name,* but no effective treatment.

Against such a backdrop of experience, how does the EFIT therapist join with the client in creating what Bowlby would describe as a *safe haven alliance,* and how does the therapist structure the process to ensure ongoing safety, the fundamental requisite for exploration and reclamation? How does the therapist tune in and find focus, then intervene in a manner that moves clients toward their leading edge of discovery but not beyond, neither overshooting nor undershooting their current capacity?

Ongoing assessment guides intervention in initial sessions and beyond. We offer a set of 10 key concepts that guide assessment/understanding and intervention, followed by transcripts and commentary featuring Sierra that illustrate the application of these core concepts and her growth through the EFIT three-stage process.

TEN KEY CONCEPTS THAT GUIDE ASSESSMENT, UNDERSTANDING, AND INTERVENTION

1. *The attachment view of health offers a benchmark and a beacon.* The image of health offered by attachment science—a felt sense of security with self and others, characterized by the capacity to (1) tune into inner emotional experience, (2) share that experience (e.g., needs, fears, longings, vulnerability) directly and coherently with key trusted others, and (3) give and (4) receive love and care—offers a benchmark by which to compare the client's present functioning, as well as a set of health indicators for assessing progress, maintaining focus, and guiding interventions toward secure attachment as therapy unfolds. Attachment security, as viewed on a continuum, offers the therapist a beacon and benchmark at outset, and throughout the therapy process.

2. *Attachment informs our understanding of the potential impacts of trauma.* Bowlby's view of healthy working models of self and other as flexible, adaptive protocols subject to ongoing revision and change in light of new, meaningful emotional and relational experiences is consistent with the developmental perspective that health is the ability to constantly adapt and grow, and that the self is ever evolving toward more depth, complexity, and coherence. In the face of intolerable stress or trauma, and the availability of a reliably safe other, there is opportunity to move with and through emotion, to even grow from such experience (e.g., see Bonanno et al., 2006). However, when trauma is consistently faced alone, blocks to growth are the inevitable consequence, primarily due to reactive intensification and/or numbing of emotion, and, over time, by extension, insecure attachment. As alluded to earlier in this book and described in greater detail elsewhere, attachment security is associated with a variety of positive health outcomes, whereas insecure attachment has been linked with a general vulnerability to mental health issues (see Johnson, 2019, for a more comprehensive overview). "From an attachment point of view, ongoing personality development involves the structuring of habitual emotional regulation strategies or styles that become especially pertinent under conditions of threat or uncertainty; the formation of a number of "hot" existential meaning frames (e.g., emotionally loaded expectations and causal attributions) that mesh with and arise from working models of self and other; and, the creation of a behavioral repertoire and specific protocols for engaging with others. These developmental processes are highly interactive and are always colored by our felt sense of [secure or insecure] connection with others" (Johnson, 2019, p. 74).

With this image of health and understanding of growth in mind, a central goal of an attachment-based experiential assessment is to iden-tify clients' vulnerabilities and strengths and the key factors and piv-otal emotional and relational experiences that have restricted or blocked growth, as well as those that have promoted resilience.

3. *Developmental considerations offer a guide to understanding and intervention.* A developmental frame guides understanding of the origins of prototypical ways of being and behaving and their develop-mental trajectory. Key from an attachment point of view is when the trauma occurred (at what age), how long it lasted, whether there was more than one traumatic event, and whether there was anyone to rely on. If growth is thwarted early in development, it follows that later devel-opmental tasks might be impacted. It also follows that if strategies for managing trauma are developed early in life with little to no reprieve in the arms of a safe attachment figure or other relevant personal or interpersonal resource, more rigid and negative models of self and other can be anticipated, as well as more automatic and reflexive affect regula-tion strategies. As viewed on a continuum, clients' reactions might range from being highly automatic and rigid (akin to a narrow window of tolerance or limited capacity), to more flexible and adaptive. From an attachment point of view, flexibility and adaptation are more likely if personal or contextual factors offer some type of refuge or resource in the face of intolerable stress or trauma. An example of this is the iden-tification and illumination of relational resources, such as a supportive other, or specific strengths.

4. *The therapist maintains a nonpathologizing stance.* In an attachment-based experiential assessment, the EFIT therapist looks at and past diagnosis at the underlying explanatory and descriptive fac-tors that inform the symptom picture. Of import is not only the surface clinical picture, but also the core self and emotional and relational pat-terns involved in the development and maintenance of that symptom picture, that is, attachment. Without attention to these self-perpetuating underlying features, change is limited and superficial—at best, achieving first-order change as described in earlier chapters, and at worst, leaving clients feeling unseen and unheard.

The therapist seeks to understand the rationality, not the pathol-ogy. Bowlby himself suggested that, in general, "clinical conditions are best understood as disordered versions of what is otherwise a healthy response" (1980, p. 245). Withdrawal and immobilization can be a func-tional response to impossible or dangerous situations where vulnerabil-ity is overwhelming (Porges, 2011), such as finding oneself dependent on an unsafe and unpredictable attachment figure. Easily triggered anger and hypervigilance are likewise adaptive when the alternative appears to be that one is inevitably dismissed or deserted. Blocks to growth occur when such responses become generalized, global, automatic, and reflexive, and thereby resistant to revision.

In initial sessions then, rather than tuning into more global constructs such as depression, the therapist focuses on the underlying structure of the client's lived emotional and relational experience. Bowlby indicated that constructs such as depression could be defined more specifically in terms of key elements. As noted earlier, he observed that depressed individuals commonly describe themselves and their lived experience in terms of four adjectives: lonely, unlovable, unwanted, and helpless (see also Johnson, 2019, for a more comprehensive review). David Barlow's unified protocol model for emotional disorders similarly looks beyond traditional diagnostic nomenclature and recognizes the overlap between various disorders such as anxiety and depression, as well as their common structure (Barlow et al., 2011). He suggests that anxiety and depression can be combined into one joint category, namely, *negative emotional disorder.* He, too, identifies common elements of various disorders such as anxiety (e.g., frequent and intense negative emotion, hypervigilance, avoidant strategies, heightened sense of threat or danger, fear of fear itself) and depression (e.g., vigilance to failure, self-criticism, social withdrawal, sense of hopelessness, and loss of motivation). These core elements are also common to trauma- and stressor-related disorders, along with elements such as intrusive and other symptoms (e.g., flashbacks, nightmares, dissociation).

When these core elements, as well as other aspects of the client's lived experience and behavior are viewed through a compassionate, survival-focused attachment lens, they will always be viewed as *reasonable*—to make sense in context. Working from that mindset, the natural focus is on following each client's pain, tuning into the way they describe themselves and their experience (i.e., the emotional handles—words, phrases, metaphors—that they use), making it tangible and making explicit the blocks to positive functioning clients unwittingly maintain or allow to overwhelm them. The aim is to understand how a particular client's natural propensity to grow and adapt has become constricted and led to self-perpetuating patterns that maintain and exacerbate symptoms of distress. Once again, however, the target of change becomes not the symptoms, but instead, the reciprocally influential and self-sustaining underlying attachment-based factors. It is understood that the natural consequence of change at this core level will extend beyond the resolution of symptoms. As well, in the face of future trauma or heightened stress, increased security will afford clients increased capacity to manage their symptoms and more readily regain their emotional balance, that is, resilience.

5. *Symptoms are at least partially understood as manifestations of attachment insecurity.* Building on the above, from an attachment point of view, symptoms are at least partially understood as the by-product of either reactive intensification or suppression of emotion and associated attributions and behavioral responses (core underlying features of attachment). Whatever the preferred method, such coping strategies are understood to create distance, from self and experience. Given the overarching goal of helping clients come home to themselves and their experience, the focus becomes proximity to self and experience, rather than symptom resolution or management. Proximity offers an initial benchmark, and a means of monitoring progress. It is anticipated that as distance shrinks, symptoms resolve.

6. *Present process links past and future.* As the EFIT therapist joins with clients in initial sessions, the focus is on *present process*. We assume that the past comes alive in the present. Initial sessions are aimed at exploring how this person is constrained by their patterns of processing experience and ways of relating with others. As the therapist tracks and reflects present process, weaving in key elements of the client's narrative and contextual factors, habitual ways of being and behaving are validated and framed in a compassionate light. Validation offers a form of psychoeducation and a means of helping clients feel seen and heard and begin to see and know themselves in new ways through a lens of compassion. Though commonly refuted in initial sessions given dominant views of self, these methods of tracking, reflection, and validation are aimed at highlighting and beginning to challenge prevailing patterns and perspectives such as self-blame.

7. *The therapist tunes in and stays attuned with CARE.* At the outset, and throughout the therapeutic process, the therapist joins with the client with CARE, that is, with attention to the dimensions of *Context, Attachment,* the *Relationship* (Therapeutic Alliance), and *Emotion* (Johnson & Campbell, 2022). A brief description of these four dimensions follows.

Context

Context refers to the importance of joining clients with attention to the context in which they live and have lived, including the broader and deeper sociocultural and intergenerational contexts. The EFIT therapist seeks to enter the phenomenological world of the client, to immerse themselves in the client's context with a stance of curiosity and humility, authenticity, and openness. Attention is given to factors such as identity (e.g., race, ethnicity, spirituality, religion, sexuality, and gender) and environment (e.g., socioeconomic, work/organizational, neighborhood), as well as experiences such as racism, sexism, ableism, and discrimination. From an attuned vantage point, the attachment lens is narrowed and widened as the EFIT therapist seeks to focus on specific aspects of the client's narrative that have likely been instrumental in shaping their view of self and other, as well as the broader landscape that inevitably has had (and perhaps continues to have) influence. Good listening on the part of the therapist is not enough. Rather, the therapist seeks full visceral and emotional engagement with the world of the client such that as the therapist sees, hears, and feels what the client is seeing, hearing, and feeling while pivotal experiences and related scenes are described, distance between therapist and client shrinks and understanding broadens. As both client and therapist deepen their understanding of the role of current and historical contextual factors in either restricting or facilitating growth, a path for further exploration is forged, along with a space for increased compassion.

Attachment

Related to *context,* the therapist endeavors to understand the developmental and relationship (*attachment*) history of the client, taking special note of what clients say about themselves and others, and how they tune into and share (or do not share) their inner emotional worlds. As viewed on a continuum, attachment security is explored as attachment strategy and capacity is discovered, along with flexibility and/or automaticity. More flexible coping and adaptation in light of new meaningful emotional and relational experiences is associated with greater attachment security, whereas a more narrow capacity, *window of tolerance,* is linked with more reflexive and automatic strategies known to restrict affect regulation and create distance between self and experience. Possible current (e.g., positive intimate relationship) and other relationship resources (e.g., spiritual figure, deceased secure attachment figure), as well as risk/vulnerability (e.g., longstanding and severe family history of depression, suicidal ideation or attempts, attachment injuries or betrayals) and resiliency factors (e.g., experiences and feelings of competence in specific areas) are explored and identified.

Coherence of narrative also is noted by the therapist, along with gaps in the client's story. In the case of incoherence and gaps, the therapist reflects and validates with a developmental frame, helping anchor and order the client's experience without concern for gaps (recognizing that they are indications of natural blocks to processing in the face of isolation and overwhelm).

Relationship

Relationship, specifically the *therapeutic alliance,* is the clinical priority and foundational in all therapies, but is especially key in EFIT and particularly when working with trauma. For individuals who have never experienced safety in relationship, this alone can be a corrective emotional experience. Once again, sensitive attunement, careful pacing, curiosity, and cultural humility guide initial sessions, both in pacing the demands of the session (e.g., the type and number of inquiries) and guiding the empathic distance of the therapist (e.g., degree to which the therapist uses voice tone and other aspects of self as an instrument in the process to guide the client into deeper levels of discovery). Difficulties with trust are common when working with trauma, and so, anticipated, as are possible ruptures. A strong therapeutic alliance is first established, then monitored, with any emerging concerns addressed (more to follow below).

Emotion

Emotion is at the center of experience and is central to EFIT. As viewed through an attachment-based lens, the therapist looks at and past diagnosis at the core and often overlapping features of emotional disorders such as heightened anxiety, hypervigilance, sad/low mood. Continuing to focus that lens, the therapist tunes into not only what is said as clients share their stories, but how it is said. The therapist tracks and attends to the way emotion is expressed (or not expressed, in the case of numbing or detachment), as well as the way emotion is regulated (e.g., anxious, avoidant, a combination of both). Specific process elements, such as body language or facial cues, voice tone, and any shifts or incongruencies, are noted as the client talks about various content areas (e.g., a tone of anger while describing an event likely to have evoked helplessness). As the therapist continually tracks and finds focus, narrowing the lens and gaining greater specificity, poignant words or phrases, images, or metaphors that represent the client's inner felt experience, that is, *emotional handles,* are bookmarked with the understanding that they might later be used to open the door to core vulnerabilities.

8. *The therapy process is structured and paced with ongoing attention to capacity.* The process and content variables outlined above, directly linked to attachment, provide the therapist with a guide to structuring and *pacing* the therapeutic process. *Accurate and on-target reflections* help clients feel seen and heard and soothe the nervous system. A

message of *collaboration* shrinks distance between client and therapist and builds trust and commitment to the process. Finally, from initial contact, and woven throughout the process, is *empathic attunement*.

The Acronym PACE

For ease of reference, and to draw attention to what is central to establishing and maintaining safety and a safe haven alliance, we offer the acronym PACE: Pacing; Accurate and on-target reflections; Collaborative process; and, Empathic attunement.

Pacing is directly linked to capacity. Capacity, or window of tolerance, is likely to vary throughout the therapeutic process, shrinking and expanding based on stress levels, exposure to trauma, processing, and/ or engaging in various means of self-care. In addition to tuning into various process elements, the therapist is attuned to possible risk factors (described in greater detail below). The central guiding question is "Can the client manage what the EFIT process demands, and at what pace?" The EFIT therapist tunes into capacity at the outset of therapy, checks in at the beginning of every session, and adjusts interventions and engagement (e.g., curiosity and exploration versus consolidation and integration) accordingly. Much like a guest in the home of another, and especially when entering the phenomenological world of the other in initial sessions, the therapist pays attention to cultural, personal, and other factors that might guide etiquette and pacing.

Accurate and on-target reflections can be, according to Rogers, revelations. Having said that, a revelation is only revelatory when the client is ready to see, hear, and integrate what is provided in the mirror the therapist is holding. As such, the therapist tunes into and stays attuned to various process elements as described above and titrates interventions (including basic reflections) accordingly. For example, at the outset of therapy, when a client's prototypical response is reflected in a tone of agitation, impatience, and irritability, though it will undoubtedly be helpful later to increase awareness of such tendencies with the overall aim of promoting flexibility and agility in response, such reflections are not likely to be welcomed in the absence of a trusting and solid therapeutic alliance. As clients feel seen and heard, in the context of a safe haven alliance, they will begin to see and hear themselves in new ways. Safety promotes exploration. Exploration facilitates growth.

Collaborative process refers to the EFIT therapist consistently, deliberately, and in various ways sending messages of collaboration to the client at the outset and throughout the process of therapy. The client's goals, commitment, and availability for therapy are noted with practicalities also considered (e.g., child care, finances, work/educational commitments) and the process is structured accordingly. The therapist joins with the client as a process consultant, guide, and safe other, not a distant expert and diagnostician (though, of course, the therapist has expertise, and this guides the process, especially early in therapy). At various points in the process, the therapist will check with the client surrounding their perceptions and experience of therapy. The goal of interventions will often be made explicit (e.g., to allow the client to feel what was intolerable, unsafe, or unacceptable to feel at the time of the event, and not alone, as nobody encounters vulnerability alone).

Empathic attunement is woven throughout the therapeutic process and is the key ingredient for safety. The above are necessary, but not sufficient conditions for the establishment of safety and maintenance of a safe haven alliance. That is, the capacity to put aside assumptions, expectations, and beliefs, and instead, fully joining with the client in the context in which they live and have lived, facilitates empathic attunement. Active listening is not enough. Rather, the EFIT therapist endeavors to get a visceral sense of the client's experience, to feel, see, touch, to know their experience through their eyes, and their felt sense. As the therapist joins with their full being, they might be moved by the client and either implicitly or explicitly express this or draw attention to specific process elements. For example, constricted breathing on the part of the client might be felt by the therapist, offering a cue to invite the client to breathe, and for the therapist to say, and "I'll breathe too," communicating to the client that they are not alone in this process of discovery and opening both to a deeper experience.

Consistent with the notion of a "good enough parent," the therapist is connected, but separate, tuning in and responding to distress, while not being overwhelmed by it. Much like how the child's tantrum in the grocery line might represent fatigue or hunger, the EFIT therapist understands that surface emotions such as frustration, agitation, and irritability may represent a version of reactive anger, overwhelm, and/or underlying anxiety. The EFIT therapist seeks to bypass the prefrontal cortex and these surface emotions and speak directly to lower parts of the brain, the seat of emotion, and the area where impacts of trauma are embedded. At times, however, and understandably, the therapist might be triggered by such surface emotions, or by anger, exasperation, or frustration more generally, even when such emotions represent deeper, more primary experience. The therapist tunes into the felt impact of such emotions, finds their own emotional balance, and responds from a place of empathy. Some clients, for example, might arrive angry, frustrated by the traffic they had just encountered or with the parking situation. For others, anger is a prototypical and reliable response, a survival mechanism to keep people at a safe distance. In some cases, the client might be highly anxious about initiating therapy and potentially exploring uncharted territory.

Whatever the circumstance, therapists use an attachment frame and a tone of empathy to respond. For example, "I am sorry parking was difficult today. I am told a nearby office is having an open house. Staff had informed clients but had not anticipated early arrivals. We apologize." At other times, especially when the anger is likely a protective strategy or prototypical way of coping, depending on intent and anticipated outcome, the therapist might take note but not speak to it directly. In other cases, validation will offer the client a means of feeling seen and heard, and their anger understood as legitimate. If underlying anxiety is perceived as central to agitation and irritability, then the therapist might say something akin to, "I recognize that I am a new person and that this might be a different experience for you. If there is anything I can do to make this more comfortable, I am very open to working with you to ensure you feel as comfortable as is possible." Again, attunement and pacing guide intervention.

9. *Ongoing assessment guides intervention.* At therapy outset and connected to the elements of PACE as described above, are various risk factors and potential contraindications for therapy. Factors such as a known and pervasive history of depression or bipolar disorder among family members, or indications of psychotic features are considered. Self-harm behaviors such as active substance abuse, disordered patterns of eating, suicidal ideation and attempts are all viewed as indications of overwhelmed social resources and systems of coping, and a possible sign that additional treatment or other resources might need to be mobilized. For example, if a reliable partner or family member is available, emotionally focused couple therapy (EFCT) or emotionally focused family therapy (EFFT) might be recommended. In other circumstances, interventions aimed at addressing various symptoms (e.g., alcohol abuse) might be introduced, either prior (e.g., in-patient rehabilitation) or concurrent (e.g., psychiatric consultation to consider medication) to a course of EFIT. In short, as the EFIT therapist joins with the client, careful attention is given to the client's capacity to manage what the EFIT clinician is likely to ask of the individual, given the client's current personal and relational resources.

With safety and a safe haven alliance prioritized, and with the goal of attachment security held at the forefront, the therapist uses the EFIT Tango to propel clients forward through the three-stage process. Initial sessions aimed at helping the therapist tune in and find focus provide the understanding necessary to chart an initial case-specific route to health.

Ongoing assessment offers refinements to this chart, and similarly, continues to guide therapeutic pacing, clinical decision-making, and interventions. Assessment and treatment merge.

Ongoing assessment is important always; it is critical when working with trauma. At the outset of therapy, and throughout the therapeutic process, interventions are pitched with attention to PACE as described above and at the client's leading edge of discovery. Said differently, the therapist seeks to work at the edge of the client's capacity, not overshooting or undershooting the window of tolerance, and gradually stretching that window/capacity. As the client engages with frightening, alien, and unacceptable emotion, the frightening becomes tolerable, the alien familiar, and the unacceptable manageable. Protective and reflexive strategies become flexible, and capacity deepens and broadens. Throughout the process, attachment science and the Tango guide focus and momentum, with Moves 4 and 5 especially aiding in tracking and highlighting change. As the client's capacity continues to expand, so too, can interventions be adjusted accordingly, with the understanding that clients can manage moving into and remaining present and engaged in experience for longer periods (in Stage 2). The Tango offers a means of assessment and focus, and therapist presence and attunement guides the implementation and intensity of micro interventions.

The Tango also offers a means of structuring the session, beginning with tuning in and finding focus with Move 1, then moving to assembling and/or deepening emotion (Move 2) and choreographing corrective emotional experiences (Move 3), then zooming out again to reflect on the process, gauge progress, and assess proximity to secure attachment (Move 4). Any shifts toward the principal goal of secure attachment, typified by the capacity to tune into one's internal emotional world, coherently share that inner experience with trusted others, and give and receive love and care, is noted. Finally, Move 5 offers a means of consolidating and highlighting gains, ongoing blocks, and future directions, as well as grounding the client and transitioning out of session. Growth occurs when clients move into and share their experience (Moves 2 and 3) whereas gains are consolidated and integrated in Moves 4 and 5. Move 1 offers opportunity to focus the session, again highlight gains, and more generally anchor the process across the three stages.

10. *Client strengths and resources are illuminated.* As the therapist joins with the client as a process consultant and temporary attachment figure, and the client provides a window into their personal and relational experiences, the therapist searches for strengths and relationships that might be resources in the therapeutic process. For example, Henny

tells us she was an elite athlete, a gymnast. These experiences of confidence and competence were a refuge from the abuse and trauma she experienced in the family home. As the therapist joins with her in the familiar gymnasium, her coach nearby, and her body perfectly poised on the balance beam, shared details begin to take Henny deep into the felt experience, an experience of acceptance and exhilaration that she can now readily access at various points in the therapy process.

ASSESSING AND INTERVENING
THROUGH THE THREE-STAGE PROCESS

We now turn our attention again to Sierra. Guided by the above principles and the map of attachment, we demonstrate how the EFIT therapist uses the Tango to propel the client through the three stages of EFT therapy, continually gauging capacity and intervening accordingly. We begin with initial sessions, then move to later sessions in Stage 1 to illustrate shifts in capacity as the client begins to engage with frightening, alien, and unacceptable emotion. Session transcripts focused on Stages 2 and 3 follow. The transcript excerpt (edited slightly for brevity) from Session 3 below offers a sample of how the EFIT therapist explores, identifies, and then illuminates a principal resource for Sierra. It also illustrates an approach to joining with the client akin to what experiential therapists denote as "entering the phenomenological world of the client." That is, walking with them into their experience, rather than hearing about and evaluating it from an expert distance. Instead of gaining access to our clients' stories through questions and answers, a checklist of symptoms, or a more comprehensive review of the multiple DSM diagnoses she has already been given, the aim is to join with Sierra as she more deeply explores the experiences that have lived in the recesses of her consciousness and continue to impact her day-to-day living. The rich details garnered through this more attachment-based experiential method of *assessment* provide both therapist and client with a deeper, more visceral understanding of the pivotal experiences, factors, and key others who have been instrumental in shaping the way Sierra sees herself, manages her inner emotional world, and impacts her interactions with and ability to trust others.

Initial Sessions with Sierra

Sierra's account of her developmental and relational history in the first two sessions was generally clear and coherent. She described her parents as descendants of survivors of residential schools, carriers of the impacts of intergenerational trauma, of told and untold stories. Descriptions of her own early childhood experiences were characterized by neglect and deprivation. Referencing the first of many diagnoses applied over the years, she described herself as "a disabled kid" living on "an inner-city reserve" oppressed by the surrounding dominant culture. Following that experience, and by then also the child of divorce, she lost interest in school and instead found refuge in the sense of belonging she felt with a small group of boys. Together, at about age nine, they discovered the analgesic effects of drugs and alcohol. Adolescent and young adult years were marked by abuse, loss, and trauma, and by ongoing addiction to drugs and alcohol. Despite this early diagnosis, however, and accompanying set of self-perceptions, she later discovered her intellect and pursued postsecondary education.

Exploration of her experience in Session 3 begins with curiosity about Sierra's earlier reference to what she described as her "inner child."

THERAPIST: Sierra, when you describe your "inner child" what do you see? What's the image that comes up for you when you use that term?

SIERRA: Well, several things. There are two images. One is alone, dark, empty, waiting, neglected. I remember being starving as a child. I remember the smell of outside, and pot and beer. I was always frightened and then I just got used to the fear. [Emotional handles such as "dark, empty, waiting, neglected, starving" poignantly capture Sierra's experience.] And then there's this other image that I have that I've only developed recently: I'm happy. I feel heard and important and taken care of and respected, appreciated. [Early in the therapeutic process, with attention to pacing, and noting elements of secure attachment, the therapist chooses to focus on this latter image, a potential resource.]

THERAPIST: How old are you in that image? The latter image, the second image?

SIERRA: Four.

THERAPIST: Oh, you're four, is that with your mom's friend?

SIERRA: Yeah, and my grandma, because my grandma circumstantially took me from my parents for a while, but I went back when I was about five or six and that's when things got really bad. [Another decision point. Again, the therapist chooses to maintain focus rather than inquiring about her phrase, "things got really bad."]

THERAPIST: So, Sierra, maybe sit with me as that little girl and help me to see your grandma, what do you see? [As a key other that can be brought to mind, Sierra's grandma might be a resource in the therapeutic process. The therapist continues to focus the session on her grandmother with the aim of evoking and further enlivening Sierra's image of her grandmother. Bringing this image to life provides a rich source of information about the security of this relationship and the potential opportunity to resource Sierra with a key attachment figure for the therapy process ahead, as well as more explicitly in her life outside therapy.]

SIERRA: My grandma? She has really dark skin and black hair, and she had worked her entire life, so she had really rough hands, but gentle at the same time, and she always wore a kerchief.

THERAPIST: What color? [As we become curious about our clients and their experiences, so too do they become curious about themselves. Over time, as details are provided, fuzzy images and memories are made vivid, the scene or person comes alive, and deeper levels of engagement with experience are reached. Past tense becomes present process. As the client becomes absorbed in their experience, protective strategies give way to increased exploration and discovery, allowing for not only information and understanding, but also a deep visceral felt sense, for both therapist and client.]

SIERRA: I have it in my room. (*Smiling.*) It's a floral print.

THERAPIST: Do you? (*Also smiling.*)

SIERRA: She had black, green, yellow, red . . .

THERAPIST: Oh, she had many colors?

SIERRA: Yeah, red was the main one, though, and she used to wear this apron all the time. And we had an orchard and a vegetable garden. And my grandpa used to go fishing all the time, so she was always gutting fish, which I thought was disgusting, but she said it's part of life. (*Now smiling again, her expression more animated and her eyes twinkling.*)

THERAPIST: Do you see her eyes? [Reframed through the lens of attachment, the therapist is actually asking, "Can you make contact with her?" but does not ask it as such, instead keeping it simple and concrete.]

SIERRA: Yeah, I do. She read to me all the time, in our Coast Salish Indigenous language. That was her first language, not English, and she sang traditional songs.

THERAPIST: How wonderful!

SIERRA: Songs for children. I had twenty-two cousins. She had no problem having us all there. She had a clothesline. My grandpa built the entire house with his brother. They had a clothesline and there were always clothes on it, and we used to run through it all the time. (*Smiling, looking off into the distance; quiet laughter.*)

THERAPIST: Oh fun! That's a beautiful image.

SIERRA: She had a huge field for her property, and me and my 22 cousins would be out there. My grandma and grandpa had nine kids. They got married when they were 21 years old. I would stay there for long periods of time, I didn't know why, but now I know why. It's because my parents were drinking and using drugs. My grandma didn't drink or use drugs, no. She had a bedroom for me there.

THERAPIST: What was your bedroom like? [Again, inquiries are made regarding details to enliven the scene, as well as the secure attachment figure, and to get a broader and deeper sense of the world she grew up in.]

SIERRA: There was a daybed in there, and there were unicorns in there and stuffed animals.

THERAPIST: What kinds of unicorns, on the wall or toys?

SIERRA: Little glass figurines or porcelain or something. Yeah, and there were Care Bears in there too. (*Smiling.*) Those toys from the early nineties/late eighties. And she would come in there, because there were so many grandchildren, we had so many children's books, and she would read those books to me before I went to bed. I remember once, I got really sick, and she stayed with me and took care of me, and nobody did that before. (*Said with an incredulous, surprised look.*) She slept in that room with me, and she read books to me. I remember that very clearly.

THERAPIST: Sierra, that is such a beautiful image—somebody being there for you and loving you and seeing you and staying with you during a time of need, when you weren't feeling well. [The therapist reflects Sierra's experience of a felt sense of security during a time of need, bringing to the forefront this "island of security" in a sea of deprivation.]

SIERRA: Yeah, and I'd never experienced that before. I'd get sick and my parents would send me to school, and I was hungry a lot because my parents were always drinking, packing me a lunch was not on their agenda. At my grandma's house, I could eat whatever I wanted. Yeah, and she had this drawer. We were all short, we were all little kids. Actually it was a cupboard, and up in that cupboard, she had all these old Coast Salish baskets, weaved baskets for salmon and berries, and that was how she was taught to cook instead of using pots and pans, and behind those baskets—my grandma didn't eat junk food, she didn't have fast food or anything or pop, but she liked candy—she would hide it from us behind those baskets and we would boost each other up to the cupboard to get the candy. (*Smiling and quietly laughing.*) [Sierra's eyes appear absorbed in the scene, as though she is back in these moments, enjoying candy with her cousins and a felt sense of security in the home and garden of her grandparents.]

As noted previously, early in the therapeutic process and with the goal of further exploring and accessing resources, the therapist chooses to focus on the more positive image. And so, Sierra's grandma comes to life. The details of her hands, the scent of her clothes, and the warmth of her embrace facilitate easy access to her grandmother, both within and outside the therapy process. With the felt sense of this relationship made more vivid, Sierra can more explicitly and deliberately rely on her grandmother as a symbolic source of security (Mikulincer & Shaver, 2004, 2013) and the therapist can readily evoke the felt experience of safety by drawing attention to specific details, such as her hands, her kerchief, and/or her loving eyes. Noteworthy, as well, is how much information this walk into her grandmother's garden provides—indications of access to culture and language, of an island of security during a time of need, and of moments of joy with her many cousins as a small child—a stark contrast to the more pervasive picture of darkness and despair provided in earlier sessions.

This provides a glimpse into the attachment-based experiential assessment, joining with clients in the worlds in which they live and have lived, and entering their worlds fully and completely to get a felt sense, a visceral understanding, more than a collection of memories, or a cognitive summary. This is always important, but especially relevant when working with trauma, when many clients do not have full access to images or memories of themselves or their experiences. As explained elsewhere, the goal of successful trauma therapy is not recovery of memory, but instead recovery of self, a more expanded, coherent, and integrated sense of self. A sense of self that can be confident in and trust internal experiences, share those internal experiences coherently and directly with key, trusted others, and not only give comfort and care, but also receive it and take it in. With this overarching goal and view of health in mind, this walk into her grandma's home also provides us with a sense of Sierra's capacity to notice and accept care and love from a trusted other. With a generally coherent narrative now noted, along with various resources (e.g., her intellect, her mom's close friend/her "auntie," and her grandmother) and a picture of some of the central figures who continue to live in Sierra's mind and heart, the therapist begins to revisit some of these key experiences that have shaped her, that left her with no choice but to block herself from feeling what was intolerable, unsafe, unacceptable to feel in the absence of a safe other. Mostly, she was alone. Her grandmother was, at times, in her life and other times not, and her mom's best friend left the community when Sierra was very young to pursue a healthier lifestyle. Even when there were others she might have relied on during a time of vulnerability, such as was the case when she was a young child and being sexually abused by two older boys, she could not turn to them. She thought that it was her fault, and she didn't really feel that she had anybody that she could tell. Incidents later in life, such as when at the age of 22 an older woman sexually assaulted her, further cemented her view of herself as unworthy and worthless. According to Sierra, by then she had grown accustomed to being violated. She did not understand physical intimacy; she did not value herself or her body and felt that she could not be loved.

Moving Into and Through Frightening, Alien, and Unacceptable Emotion

Turning now to later sessions in Stage 1, the therapist begins to expand capacity and create flexibility by helping Sierra move into and through what Bowlby described as frightening, alien, and unacceptable emotion. As capacity expands, so too does access/proximity to self and the possibility of a more expanded, coherent, and integrated sense of self. To begin to focus and order experience, based on the initial attachment-based experiential assessment, and using the EFIT Tango as a guide, the therapist provides a reflective summary of how Sierra organizes and manages her inner emotional world and how that plays out relationally with others (Move 1 of the Tango). This is the EFIT version of diagnosis, a reflective summary that gets to the heart of the matter, that captures the way clients organize their inner emotional worlds, how they dance with themselves and others, and how this pattern of being and relating makes sense in context, was adaptive but is now limiting.

The therapist says, "I hear you Sierra, it makes sense you would numb out and shut down, at times get angry and lash out, that was the safe thing to do. What I hear you saying is your early experiences were colored by neglect, abuse, hunger. You used the word "starvation." There was no safe space for you and your vulnerability. For their own reasons that you partially understand based on their personal and inter-generational contexts, your parents could not be there for you. You were alone. Mostly, you coped by numbing out and shutting down, shutting off emotionally and with substances, and now, what I hear you saying is that these strategies are preventing you from connecting with those you wish to connect with— your wife, but also some friends and family. You're still alone and lonely."

Sierra nods affirmatively. The therapist then draws attention to some of the key self-perpetuating aspects of this way of being and behaving, emotionally and relationally, and how these protective strategies have now become a prison. Following the opportunity for Sierra to reflect and process, the therapist shifts to Move 2 of the Tango, and explores *trigger* and *response, bodily sensation, meaning,* and *perception*—the core elements of emotion (Arnold, 1960). Sierra can readily identify the trigger as perceptions of threat (e.g., criticism, anger). Her automatic response is to recoil, shut down, get quiet, lash out in anger, or some combination of them all. As the therapist joins with Sierra in ordering her experience, both therapist and client begin to understand that any type of interpersonal discord leads to fears of abandonment. It is better to stay hidden than to risk rejection or loss. Sierra reports a lack of access to any bodily sensations. She feels numb. As the therapist invites Sierra to tune into and notice other elements, Sierra can articulate the meaning she makes—the attachment significance—of these common interactional patterns. Core phrases and/or emotional handles capture the attachment significance: "bad," "helpless," "alone," "lonely," "I'm not important," "I don't matter," and "I can't trust anyone."

In a later session, still in Stage 1 of the therapy process, Sierra identifies various memories and experiences that capture and represent themes of being alone, numb, and detached. As she gets close to that experience in her backyard, memories of her cousins, abuse, loss, trauma, the death of relatives to suicide, all rush forward. Her grandmother's garden is in eyesight but inaccessible, following "the intervention" with her mother and her mother's subsequent ban on any contact with extended family. Focusing the session, the therapist invites Sierra to stay still with her experience, rather than distancing herself from it through numbing or reactive intensification, and to focus on one of the many memories currently bombarding her.

THERAPIST: Sierra, if we stay really still in that experience, I mean, I get it, the thing that happens is that when we get close to some of these difficult moments in your life, it's like a flood of memories come back, images and fleeting pictures of people and things that have happened. But if we still the video, stop the video and just stay focused on you, and let all those other pictures fade into the background, what do you see when you see that 10-year-old? [The overall aim here is to begin to allow Sierra to feel some of what was intolerable and unsafe to feel at the time of these earlier experiences, to begin to encounter frightening, alien, and unacceptable experience, making it more tolerable, familiar, and manageable. Focusing on her younger self, rather than the deluge of memories, helps make it more manageable and facilitates a focus on one scene representative of many involving themes of abandonment, neglect, being alone and lonely, shut down, or shut off, with the understanding that accessing and processing the emotions/experience of one such scene will generalize and impact the core elements of attachment that have been shaped by these scenes/experiences that share similar themes.]

SIERRA: I used to play in the backyard by myself after school. I would walk home and nobody would be there. My sister would go to a babysitter with her best friend. Again, she had better opportunities than I did. Even though I was alone, it wasn't dangerous because my grandma's house was right there. Although my mom didn't let me talk to her during that time, she was right there. [Move 1, consistent theme of being alone and lonely.]

THERAPIST: You could feel your grandma's presence. [Reflection that draws attention to her grandmother, a key resource and source of safety.]

SIERRA: It was on her property and I knew nothing was going to happen there.

THERAPIST: Sierra, if we go into that space, and I'll come too, help me to see the backyard, is it treed or is it lawn, or is it . . . ? [Therapist communicates, "I'm here, too; you're not alone," further resourcing the client.]

SIERRA: It's rectangular, and there's a big hill and a cherry tree. There's this massive, huge tree, and there's a whole bunch of old maple trees and a lilac tree, too.

THERAPIST: What time of year is it Sierra? [Specificity facilitates manageability and brings the scene alive.]

SIERRA: Fall.

THERAPIST: Okay. So, the lilacs are gone and . . .

SIERRA: Do you know when the sun starts setting, like pretty much as soon as your workday's over, and outside is already dark?

THERAPIST: Yeah, that's where you are. It's in the fall, afterschool and before dark, but it's starting to get dark. Where is this 10-year-old girl? Where are you? [Assess proximity.]

SIERRA: We had a woodshed and we had an A-frame-like shed with the basketball hoop on the front of it. Behind it, we had a swing on a tree. I played on the swing, on the whole property.

THERAPIST: Sierra what do you feel in your body as you get close to that young 10-year-old you? [Move 2 of the Tango.]

SIERRA: I don't feel anything. [No access to frightening, alien, and unacceptable emotion.]

THERAPIST: That's okay. Are you able to get close to her? Are you able to move toward her? And I'll be with you. I can feel the yard more now.

SIERRA: Yeah, I can.

THERAPIST: Yeah? Where are you in relation to her? [Therapist continues to gauge proximity.]

SIERRA: My grandfather poured a concrete basketball court.

THERAPIST: Oh wow.

SIERRA: It was, you know, the key on the basketball court, we had that. So close but not too close, that's what I see, several feet, maybe eight feet away. [Therapist notes that proximity to self seems to be increasing as therapy progresses. At the outset of therapy, Sierra connected with her younger self from about 20 feet.]

THERAPIST: Help me to see what you see, I'll be with you, near that basketball key. It's good Sierra, you are doing a great job, stay really still in your gut. [The therapist encourages and invites Sierra to remain connected to her body, her internal world, to move into the experience, rather than talking about it, as much as she is able and at the leading edge of her capacity/within her window of tolerance.]

SIERRA: It's hard because I was so damaged already. Even with my own family, I would stay away.

THERAPIST: Right, it's hard to get close to her because she was so . . .

SIERRA: Hurt.

THERAPIST: Yeah. "Hurt." That's a good word isn't it, "hurt." [The therapist notes and prefers this descriptor over "damaged" because "hurt" captures what happened to her, rather than how she views herself.]

SIERRA: Even my own mom. . . . I would stand on the other side of the room from her, probably from that age until I was 30.

THERAPIST: Well Sierra, this is good. Okay, so she's eight feet away and you're there, and I'm there right behind you, beside you. [Resourcing the client and narrowing the focus, zooming in.] If you just stay in your body now and you see her, from eight feet away, help me to see her a bit more, what's she wearing, Sierra? So that I can really be there with you as well. [Again, details bring the experience to life and allow both therapist and client to become increasingly absorbed in it. The goal of an experiential emotionally focused therapy is to move into the experience, and in this first stage of the therapy process, to begin to access and touch the emotions associated with that experience.]

SIERRA: I don't even really remember my clothes, specifically.

THERAPIST: Okay, Sierra, maybe not from your memory but just from your body now, as you are in that scene and I'm there, too, what just comes up? It doesn't have to be accurate. What's the image that comes up for you of that 10-year-old?[Accessing more details with the goal of contacting, recovering self, not memories.]

SIERRA: Yeah. I remember my older cousins used to give me jeans, so I wore poorly fitting jeans all the time.

THERAPIST: How's your hair? What does your hair look like? What's her hair look like?

SIERRA: It was really . . . my hair was really dark, almost black during those years. Nobody even taught me how to put my hair in a pony at that age, so it was down all the time, and it wasn't, like nicely down, I would just let it go.

THERAPIST: As long hair, short, medium?

SIERRA: Like here. (Points; indicating her shoulder-length hair.) My mom used to give me these horrible haircuts, so maybe, twice a year I'd get a haircut and I just hated it, so I would look forward to growing it out until I had to get my next haircut. But I remember I went like three or four years without a haircut. [Again, therapy moves toward increased specificity and detail to enliven the scene and those within it, and to increase access to self and inner emotional world.]

THERAPIST: Sierra, this is good, let's stay in that space. I can sense the yard and the basketball hoop and the sheds and this young you, this 10-year-old in that space. You're there and I'm in your background, alongside you. You're about eight feet away and she's wearing baggy jeans and her hair's down. Do you see her face, Sierra? [Again, the therapist uses process summaries, capturing the details to create a container around the experience, to maintain focus, and to keep the therapeutic work specific and manageable.]

SIERRA: Yeah, I do.

THERAPIST: Help me to see her. What do you see when you see her face?

SIERRA: I was quite vacant. [As details are provided, increased access to self and experience is gained.] You know, if my expression wasn't vacant . . . yeah, it was fear or vacancy. [Access to and specificity of emotion is shifting from "I don't feel anything" to "vacant" to "fear or vacancy."]

THERAPIST: What do you see in her eyes now? [If accessible, the eyes provide a clear and direct window into experience.]

SIERRA: Fear. [Therapist notes increased specificity as they maintain focus; "fear or vacancy" shifts to "fear."]

THERAPIST: Yeah, okay. Good Sierra. What do you, what does your gut want to say to her, if your body could speak? [Setting up a Move 3 encounter.]

SIERRA: I'm not going to hurt you. [Therapist hears, "You are safe with me."]

THERAPIST: That's nice Sierra. What happens to her eyes when you say that? [Move 4 of the Tango, the impact on felt experience.]

SIERRA: They change.

THERAPIST: What do they look like? [Questions are open-ended and remain focused on visible, body/expression-based shifts in affect. Therapist follows rather than leads. The client is in the experience and the therapist trusts the power and potency of attachment and the safe haven space Sierra is in at this time.]

SIERRA: Relief. [Therapist notes a positive impact on felt experience.] I used to hold my breath when people would approach me. [Sierra notes the contrast between relief and holding her breath, restriction, a sign of fear, or insecurity. A small shift has been made toward secure attachment.]

THERAPIST: Is she breathing now?

SIERRA: Yeah. [Therapist hears this as a signal that Sierra is continuing to feel safe, to stay in this felt experience of security.]

THERAPIST: Yeah. Yeah. What are you drawn to do next, Sierra? Now what happens? [The EFIT therapist follows and leads. With the experience up and running and notable shifts occurring, the therapist now follows as this Move 3 encounter unfolds.]

SIERRA: Nobody asked me questions about my life. Nobody asked me what I thought or felt. [Therapist hears, "Nobody saw me." Belonging leads to becoming, that is the story of human development. As the client gains greater access to a felt sense of security, the sense of loss and no sense of belonging, comes to the forefront. At this point in the process, the therapist maintains focus on helping Sierra to feel what she was unable to feel and to access comfort from key others.]

The sense of loss that so inevitably accompanies trauma will need to be addressed later in the therapy process to make space for what key others can now provide and/or do offer in other relationships, such as with her wife.]

THERAPIST: Do you want to ask her? Do you want to ask her questions? What do you want to ask her, Sierra? [Therapist keeps the Move 3 encounter going.]

SIERRA: How are you? How are you doing?

THERAPIST: What does she say? What does she say back?

SIERRA: I used to just say "fine" all the time. "Fine." But nothing was fine, like, literally nothing. [The therapist notes that Sierra has come out of the experience slightly, now commenting in past versus present tense, as it is a memory, rather than a felt experience. Recognizing that this is a lot to manage, the therapist now shifts the Move 3 encounter and invites Sierra to be in the body of the 10-year-old.]

THERAPIST: Are you able to be in her body? Do you feel like you could be in her body? And I'll be with you. Are you able to be in her body and share? If I ask you, "How are you?" Are you able to share, from your gut, in the body of that 10-year-old, with the baggy jeans or the unfitting jeans I think you said. [More Move 2 of the Tango, deepening, and setting up Move 3 encounter.]

SIERRA: If I had to be that person, I think it would be super traumatic for me. [This is important. The therapist hears Sierra's reluctance, that she is perhaps at the far edge of her capacity/window of tolerance. Therapist responds with a rationale and an invitation to share, as she is able, within her window of capacity. The goal here, if she can manage it, is to tune into and share with a safe other what she was unable to share as a young child, a *corrective emotional experience,* an antidote to trauma.]

THERAPIST: I hear you, Sierra, that's exactly what this is all about, to be able to feel what that little girl wouldn't have felt safe to feel, and to share that with somebody, to not be alone in it. That's what this is all about but not for it to be traumatic, of course. So, you tell me how this goes, okay? [Transparency provides agency, both in terms of the goal and the assurance that it should not be traumatic, and that she can gauge/control that.] Do you feel like you can share from your gut, from your body, from your throat, from your chest, about that feeling of being alone and abandoned and hurt, not trusting? [As highlighted above, note the word "hurt" is used to highlight what happened to her, not how she views herself. The focus here is to capture her experience and begin to help her feel. Self-definition will be more explicitly addressed in Stage 2 of the model: restructuring self and system.]

SIERRA: It's so bad. Like I can't articulate. (*Now tearful and crying.*) I can't be the 10-year-old, just being there is a lot. [Therapist hears her say, "This is enough."]

THERAPIST: It's okay Sierra, I hear you, you are doing amazing. Good for you to give voice to some of that experience as much as you're able. It's good Sierra. Let yourself breathe and feel some of that. You don't have to be alone in it this time.

As Sierra breathes, opening space for herself and her experience, the therapist remains silent until it's noticeable that her affect shifts again. The therapist then uses a soft, slow voice to provide a Move 5 summary, to celebrate and consolidate gains, and to offer an opportunity for closure and transitioning out of the experience, a type of grounding following this important therapeutic work.

THERAPIST: Do you see what you just did, Sierra? Do you see what happened? (*Pause. Sierra nods and breathes.*) As you took the risk of being still with that younger you, in your yard, the safety of your grandma's garden close by, and I was there, too, in the background, you were able to get closer to your experience, the experience you would not have felt safe to feel at that time, that no young child would feel. Nobody encounters vulnerability alone. That's not how we're wired. But in the safety of your grandma's presence and that older wiser you, you were able to stay still with your experience, "nothing" shifted to "vacant," to "fear or vacancy," that's what you said, that was your core experience. And as you stayed still with you, that younger you, you found fear in her eyes, and as she felt seen, fear shifted to relief, and she could breathe, you could breathe. You didn't have to hold your breath. You recalled that no one asked you about you, your thoughts, and feelings, and you asked, "How are you?" "Fine," she said, but you knew, you know, literally, nothing was fine. And then you took an even bigger step forward, Sierra. You were able to be in the body of that young child, something you have been avoiding for a long time, for lots of good reasons, and you were able to feel and share some of the vulnerability you were previously unable to feel or share. There was no one there for you Sierra, but now there is, and as you get closer to you, like you already are—you're doing an amazing job Sierra—you are going to find more of you and your experience. That's how this works, Sierra, the more that you can find and be closer to you, the more you can share your inner world with others, the closer you can be to those you trust. You will still be able to hide or shut down. You can choose when and who you trust. You're doing beautiful work, Sierra. Good for you.

As Sierra sits in silence, seemingly processing all of this, the therapist checks in with her.

THERAPIST: Sierra, what was it like for you to reconnect with that younger you, and share some of those feelings?

SIERRA: It's not as bad as I thought it would be. I avoid talking about those years as much as I possibly can.

THERAPIST: What do you feel now that you have?

SIERRA: I don't know if "liberated" is, it's not the right word, but that part of me was so silenced.

The therapist reflects that which they want the client to notice, as viewed through the lens of attachment and with an eye on the goal: a felt sense of security with self and others. The above Move 5 summary highlights shifts in affect and proximity to self, as well as interpersonal safety and security, the core elements of attachment. It also provides Sierra with a clear roadmap for change and increased flexibility and trust in self and experience. The interactional sequence offers two corrective emotional experiences. First, Sierra finds relief in being seen. This gives her the opportunity and courage to move deeper into her felt experience and to share her vulnerability, the vulnerability she could not have felt in earlier times and could not have shared. She had no one.

The interactional sequence to follow the Move 5 summary is intended to further process the session (Move 4), to gauge capacity and Sierra's experience of the emotional demands of the session (assessment) and is an additional means of transitioning outside the therapy context. Sierra acknowledges that it was not as bad as she thought it would be, an important indicator for the therapist, suggesting it was within her window of capacity and so manageable, not traumatic. Following these comments, Sierra acknowledges that no one said these things to her, no one saw her, and she would have felt less helpless and hopeless if someone had told her that she was going to use her intellect to find her way out. With that, she is invited to share this knowing with the

10-year-old (another Move 3 encounter), and as she does so, she sees the young child's eyes shift to "super happy." At the end of the session, Sierra resolves to try to keep all those difficult memories in the background and this smiling young child and her grandmother close by, and says she is going to think about the right word for her experience; "relief," for sure, maybe "liberating," she is uncertain.

Moving forward in the therapeutic process, through Stage 1, key traumatic experiences that have shaped Sierra rise to the forefront and are recounted. A host of incidents involving themes of abuse, loss, and trauma color the landscape of Sierra's life. Once again, it is not necessary to process and choreograph corrective emotional experiences for all such events. Instead, specific scenes representative of such consistent themes are addressed with the overarching goal of restructuring attachment, challenging prevailing templates surrounding view of self and other, and broadening capacity to move with and through emotion; effective affect regulation. The goal is to increase capacity, to bring clients home to themselves. That is, to titrate interventions with sensitive attunement such that proximity/access to self increases, and frightening, alien, and unacceptable emotions become tolerable, familiar, and manageable. As the client's capacity to slow down and tune into their inner emotional world increases, the space between trigger and response widens, window of tolerance broadens, and clients can more readily find their emotional balance in moments of distress. Symptoms improve in terms of frequency and/or intensity.

With increased capacity to engage more deeply with emotion, with more coherence, and for longer periods, clients can access core vulnerabilities and key defining identity dilemmas in Stage 2. Against this backdrop of growth, Sierra reflects on the therapy process toward the end of Stage 1 and into Stage 2.

Accessing Self and Experience at Deeper Levels

SIERRA: When I started speaking with you, I think I was really in shock about everything that had happened in my life. I didn't know how to process a lot of things. Now that I've been able to step away and focus on me, everything is hitting me really hard. I'm becoming conscious of my feelings and how my life experiences, historical life experiences, shape a present perception of what's happening now. All these things happened, and it didn't bother me before because I wasn't . . . I don't feel like I was awake. Now I feel more aware of these things that have some sort of influence on my daily affairs, and as much as I enjoy it, I also dislike being aware of it. I have feelings of resentment toward people, adults mostly, who were in my life when I was a child, because I'm starting to realize the gravity of things that happened and just how easy it was for so many people to turn their back on me. And now when things happen that I don't like, I see how I get triggered and then everything's a write-off. I don't stay angry for very long now, like I did when I first met you, but now I go to sadness, and I look at myself. [Maintaining focus on the overarching goal, an expanded sense of self, and trusting that Sierra will negotiate these relationships as best for her once this central goal is achieved, the therapist gauges/assesses where they are in the process and begins to focus the session with a question about how Sierra sees herself currently.]

THERAPIST: And when you see yourself, what do you see? [Assessment and treatment merge, an intervention to focus the session, and a means of assessing current view of self based on the understanding that growth occurs within and between sessions, and a key role of the therapist is to continually assess progress and intervene to keep the client at their leading edge of growth.]

SIERRA: I'm not good enough, I'm not smart enough. I'm not nice enough. I don't make enough money. I could be in better shape. I could be a better friend. I could be a better sibling, cousin. Like nothing is good enough about me. I feel like I've missed out so much on developing as an adult because everything was chaos when I was growing up. Now that I'm really in my responsibility, I feel frustrated that I don't know how to do normal things, and then I go to, "I'm stupid." For example, the doctoral program I'm in. Obviously, you must be intelligent to get in, but I go through this whole, "I'm a fraud, I'm not like my other classmates." My teachers have expressed time and time again and directly pointed out things that I share in class, how I've helped facilitate classes and that they find my research extremely intriguing. And for some reason, I still think I don't deserve to be in the program. [View of self is at the forefront, undeserving, unable to take in care and respect from others, a key element of secure attachment.]

THERAPIST: You don't take any of that in, it's hard for you to take any of that in, is that right? [Block is reflected.]

SIERRA: That's right and what I see, you know what comes to my mind, the front of my mind, is my dad's new wife saying that I have no personality, and then I think everything that I've ever done is fake. [A key identity-defining experience, again representative of many such experiences with similar themes.]

THERAPIST: Sierra, do you see the little girl that she was speaking to, that young girl?

SIERRA: Yeah, yeah.

THERAPIST: What do you see when you find you in that space?

SIERRA: I remember being frozen. I didn't know how to interpret that. I was about six. Like, does that mean I'm not, like I remember thinking, does that mean I'm not a person? And then I started to question the way I saw myself, because what she saw and what I felt about me were completely different. I also felt like I had no value or purpose, although back then, I couldn't express that's how I felt. I don't even think I could say that I felt worthless because I didn't know how to express that. But now when I look back, I can put words to the feeling, and I find that I still feel that way. [The past comes alive in the present. That is, key defining identity dilemmas that have shaped view of self actively influence present views of self and interactional patterns. As therapy progresses and clients transition from Stage 1 into Stage 2 with greater capacity and increased access to self and self-definition, the Tango can more explicitly and deliberately be used to reshape self and self-definition. The therapist is attentive to Sierra's insight and ability to articulate her view of self as "worthless" and recognizes that with her increased capacity, they can likely begin to more explicitly restructure self and system.]

THERAPIST: Sierra, are you able to get close to her, that little 6-year-old in this space, that frozen little girl, are you able to do that? Are you able to get near her and I'll be here, too, of course, in the ways that we've done in the past? [It is recognized that Sierra now has a template for the structure of the session; she knows how to dance the Tango.]

SIERRA: I think so. I can try. I remember not feeling scared in that moment. I was like, "What the f*** does that mean?" And I told my sister that, too. My sister was, like, three and a half and I was six. I remember that conversation.

THERAPIST: That's good, Sierra. The thing I hear you saying is that when we met, you could find anger and you lived in that quite a bit, but the place you are now, as you beautifully, poignantly, and powerfully shared, is that you feel more awake. I think you said, "I feel more aware. I feel more conscious of my feelings. I feel more, I guess, alive in a lot of ways, not so frozen." But there's a part of you that's still that little girl, that younger you who questions herself and doubts herself and is getting to know herself. So Sierra, when I take you back to that space, to be closer to you, that part of you that had to shut down, that froze to survive and then went into all kinds of other spaces to stay a long distance away from you, and from those who, at that time, were not able to be there for you and hold you and comfort you and protect you and take care of you, it's about shifting some of those impacts that you're becoming more and more aware of. So, the place I was going to go, just so that you are aware, and we don't have to do that if that's not where you are, is to tell her, what would you say to her when you see her and find her, that younger you? [Again, transparency provides agency and explicitly communicates that the therapy process is collaborative.]

SIERRA: I see exactly where I am in this situation. There was this really dark hallway at my dad's house, down at the end was this spare bedroom and I used to sleep down there, even the room was excluded from the rest of the house. [Another poignant image of no sense of inclusion, of belonging.] I remember standing in that dark hallway because nobody ever went down there, and if I needed to remove myself from the situation at my dad's house, sometimes I would just really miss my mom when I was there, I would go stand in that dark hallway, and that's where I am when I'm thinking of myself right now, as a kid.

With this core defining identity dilemma now at the forefront and the scene made vivid (Move 1 of the Tango), Sierra is now in a better position to feel what would have been unsafe, intolerable, and unmanageable to feel for any 6-year-old. Sierra explains that her older, wiser adult self is now able to get close to her, "right beside her." The immediate response from this 6-year-old is relief, "a safe person." Again noting that as proximity to self has increased over the past sessions along with trust, the therapist then asks, "What are you drawn to do, Sierra, as you get that close and tune into her relief and her sense of safety?"

SIERRA: I want to nurture that kid, comfort that kid, but I can see that child doesn't necessarily want to be touched or hugged, doesn't know how to accept it. [The attachment map and view of self as a guide to assessment and intervention, the therapist recognizes that Sierra is still unable to fully take in care and love from others, a key element of secure attachment.]

THERAPIST: You could talk to her about that or just even communicate, however that might look between you, and I'll just stay, I'll stay a little further away but be there, too. [Again, resourcing the client, as older wiser Sierra is invited to share with her younger self in this key defining identity dilemma, what she sees and hears, and/or how she might respond to what she sees and hears.]

SIERRA: I'm saying to this kid, "Don't listen to her. You're a great kid, you have personality. She doesn't know who you are. Do not listen to her." [As the scene is made vivid and Sierra is readily absorbed in the experience, she can directly and coherently challenge these words that have impacted her and been instrumental in shaping her view of herself—Move 3 of the Tango.]

THERAPIST: And then what happens?

SIERRA: The child is listening.

THERAPIST: Sierra, does she take it in? [Move 4 of the Tango and, as noted above, a means of assessing impact within session, as well as beginning to highlight any shifts toward attachment security.]

SIERRA: Yes.

As the session progresses and Sierra stays in her experience, her core vulnerability, she witnesses and is connected to the tears of the young child, her younger self. When asked what she is drawn to do (Move 3 of the Tango), Sierra says to the young child, the younger version of herself, "I'm sorry you're the one who's bearing the brunt of the abuse." Self-blame and self-deprecation, and feelings of worthlessness and being undeserving, shift to self-compassion. View of self is being challenged at deeper levels of experience, a central goal in EFIT.

THERAPIST: What happens to her little face when you say that? [Move 4 of the Tango.]

SIERRA: She's very upset. [Affect deepens.]

THERAPIST: What's happening inside of you Sierra?

SIERRA: I actually feel like, for once, an adult could see what was going on and acknowledge it. I can see that the child is in pain, but I don't feel that same pain myself right now. But also, part of why the child version of me is crying is because I feel seen for the first time in a long time. I only felt that with my grandma and my mom's friend, and when my mom was sober. So, to tell myself that in this situation, the tears that I'm seeing, that this child has, are because she feels seen, I feel seen, and even though I'm not saying anything, I feel heard. [She feels seen and heard, another corrective emotional experience.]

THERAPIST: That's nice, Sierra. So now as you breathe and stay in this space, what are you drawn to do? What's next? What feels right for you? [Therapist follows, rather than leads, as the Move 3 encounter and felt experience continues to take hold.]

SIERRA: Now I have this whole scenario that never happened. I wanted to charge around the corner and snatch the phone from my dad's wife and call my mom to go home that morning. When I drank and did drugs, I used to imagine that really happening, but it didn't happen because I was so shocked.

THERAPIST: Of course, Sierra. What happens now? What happens for you now, in this moment, for that little girl and for you in that space, and I'm down the hall and close by. [Maintaining momentum, keeping the experience alive.]

SIERRA: I still don't want to be touched, but I do ask the adult version of myself to go home. [Now fully connected to the felt experience that she has previously been unable to feel in the context of this key event and in the presence and safety of a reliable attachment figure, Sierra can now tune into her needs and express them, coherently and directly, a core element of secure attachment.]

THERAPIST: Okay, good. Now what? [Once again, with the experience up and running, the therapist follows rather than leads.]

SIERRA: I'm grabbing the bags, grabbing my sister and leaving. I don't even care to say goodbye to my dad. I was so set on hiding these things from my mom because I didn't want to make her more angry. [This need is met. Sierra finds her agency.]

THERAPIST: You were protecting, not protected. [Therapist reflects with a focus on the attachment significance.]

SIERRA: I want to go home and tell my mom. [She is seen and heard, trauma is being transformed, and Sierra finds her agency—a solution to her vulnerability—she finds a solution to her vulnerability through the agency she did not have, any 6-year-old child would not have, at the time of this key defining event.]

THERAPIST: Okay. I'll follow you Sierra, you lead the way. [Therapist continues to follow.]

SIERRA: I've never told my mom anything before because I never expected her to protect me. I'm hesitant to tell my mom. . . . I'm in the driveway at my mom's house. I want to tell her and I don't want to tell her. I'm sitting in this car . . . I'm sitting in my mom's old car in this scenario, the car she had when I was a kid. I won't go inside and tell her. One thing that's always made me angry about my mom is that whenever she knew about my problems, she cried more than I ever did. And we would have, maybe, one good weekend where she would be there and do things with me, and then the next weekend, she would go out and disappear, be gone. So, I learned not to tell her anything. I wouldn't tell her things because I hated the pattern, but then if I didn't tell her, I had nobody to protect me from anything.

At this point in the session, Sierra's voice is firmer and more confident, and her posture more upright, signs that trauma is transforming, and her agency is being discovered. As she sits in the driveway of her family home, her adult self in the driver's seat, she ponders whether to go inside her family home and seek the support of her mother, the support she desires and longs for but knows is highly unreliable. Instead, she drives across the bridge into the city, the same bridge she crossed as a young child with her mom's best friend, and the same bridge she crossed on her bicycle with the group of boys she befriended in middle childhood. As they cross the bridge, the young child in the backseat, Sierra acknowledges, "I felt homeless at that time, I felt that way most of my life. Now I can see how much it means to this child and how important it is for that child to trust somebody, and I see that I can be that person." The therapist notes the indications of increased compassion and a shift toward a felt sense of security.

The therapist continues to follow Sierra and this beautiful young child, this younger version of herself, across the bridge and into the city, now at the beach that was a common refuge for that young child, a place she would ride her bike and then watch other children playing and laughing on the swings. Sierra concludes, "I can hold this kid's hand when we're walking, which is something I couldn't do 10 minutes ago. And I can take her down to those swings and push her and play with her." Her fears, needs, and longings now acknowledged and attended to with a reliable and safe other, Sierra can offer a safe haven for play and exploration, the building blocks of security and growth in connection.

This is home, a felt sense of safety and security, something she mostly did not have, most certainly did not reliably have as a young child. "Kids are taught to hold the adult's hand when walking on the street and I never really had that," Sierra reflected toward the end of the session. These and other comments again remind us of the importance of grief in processing trauma. Indeed, as Sierra gets in touch with what is and can be, what could have been but was not—a felt sense of security with self and others—feelings of grief and loss naturally emerge. At this stage in the process, the therapist acknowledges and validates this as part of the natural process of moving with and through some of the emotions that would naturally be associated with a childhood devoid of so much.

Continuing to move forward as she consolidates all that has happened in this powerful session, Sierra remarks, "I feel like the real me is more visible or more there, that I am more there than I have been before because I never reconciled things in my childhood before." As progress is gauged, the therapist hears indications of the reclamation of previously disavowed aspects of self. Further assessing location in the process and using the core elements of attachment as a beacon, the therapist directly inquires about Sierra's view of self: "When you see the real you, what do you see?" Sierra replies, without hesitation, "A normal kid, happy. I'm not paranoid or anxious or scared or worried, not overwhelmed, angry, sad, crying, alone. None of those things." Increasingly liberated from the grip of trauma and its impacts, Sierra can now see and feel herself in a new light.

Final Sessions and Ongoing Shifts Toward Security

The growth process now kickstarted, Sierra continues to grow both within and between sessions over Stage 2 and into Stage 3. At one point, when asked about what she sees when she looks for herself in her current landscape as she is now, Sierra describes a field, green rolling hills, and a big sky: "Idaho in the spring." The feeling is one of hope and peace. She sees herself as her current age and hears the words, "Thank you for bringing me here." "It is a peaceful and comfortable scene," she says, smiling, as it is on the journey to becoming an elder, but the image is not permanent. She recognizes that others have also taken this journey— her grandmother and her ancestors—that she will continue to grow and learn, and that the voice of her grandmother, now more audible and ever present, will continue to guide her.

As Sierra further describes her perspective of the therapy process in later sessions, she portrays a shift in perspective. Contrasting her current experience with the outset of therapy and squinting as she squeezes her pointing finger and thumb together to create a small gap, she reflects, "You know, my lens for life was like this big." Her internal and external world now expanded, along with her ability to cope, she conveys that when she gets triggered, she is no longer the small child with her stepmother, or the lonely or disappointed young child or teen. Elaborating further regarding the shift in perspective, she adds, "I can see the change in me, toward myself and others. My perceptions of reality are changing in a good way, a positive way. I'm less angry. My stepmom, my dad, my mom, my abusers, my teachers, the police officer, everybody—they hold less of a space inside me now. It used to make me angry, knowing that my actions were almost dictated by these bad memories with these people. Their presence isn't as frequent or as heavy now. Rather than those people, the people that are in my mind, in my daily affairs, it's not people I resent anymore, it's my sister, my mom today and not my mom from 10 years ago, my grandma, my auntie." As trauma moves from the forefront to the back and perception expands beyond threat and danger, new and more positive memories emerge.

Elaborating further, Sierra states, "I feel like I've finally found my inner child. It's like the gap is closing. The distance and the darkness between me and finding myself got a little closer and a little closer and a little closer, and then this sadness, this grief, of finally coming face-to-face with a childhood that was devastating." But the best part of this, she continued, had been finding pockets of great things. Sierra recounts memories of moments of happier times with her mother, the smell of the cookies she made during periods of sobriety over the holidays, and the pride she felt when her mom greeted her in their Coast Salish language along with her classmates as they passed through the hallway into the school gym. Describing intricate details of the wooden blocks that fascinated her as a young child, Sierra is once again absorbed as she recalls the smell of them, marked with letters and primary colors. She concludes that her mom must have been doing well, "Because there's no way I would've been playing with those blocks if she was drinking or disappearing, for me to even be able to play when I was a kid, I needed to feel safe." Wise words, supported by attachment science.

As these and other experiences are recalled, and integrated into her personal narrative, the compassion she has gained for herself extends to others, affording opportunity to navigate and re-negotiate relationships with key others. Resentment and anger now in the background, she can see her mother in her intergenerational context and as a single parent, and is aware her mom holds secrets that continue to haunt her. She is grateful for the pockets of wellness her mother had and for her mother's current ability to stay healthy and have a healthy relationship with her children, be the mother Sierra longed for in earlier times. Sierra recognizes that the love and care she provides her nephews is what she now has, can take in, and was once missing. Such observations also signal grief and are a sign of the intergenerational impacts of healing. Describing herself as "stepping out of [her] trauma," Sierra again references her goal to become an elder in her community: "I want to look back on my life when I'm an elder and say, 'I lived my life by being me, my authentic self,' and maybe—I think I am—I'm on that path to becoming an elder."

PLAY AND PRACTICE

For You Personally

We are all impacted by the context in which we live and have lived, including our own intergenerational contexts. As you reflect on the landscape of your life, what key events or experiences shaped you? Who are the key characters that continue to live in your heart and mind, and how have they and do they continue to influence you? Are there resources that you can more explicitly and deliberately rely on if brought to the forefront, as was the case with Sierra's grandmother? Write out a developmental timeline that captures and summarizes these experiences and key others.

For You Professionally

If you were to describe this model to a colleague unfamiliar with EFT or the EFIT approach, what would you say? Write out what you would say about how the EFIT therapist joins with the client, tunes in, and finds focus, and so structures the therapy process. What would you say about how assessment and intervention merge throughout the therapy process?

KEY TAKEAWAYS

Ten Key Concepts of an Attachment-Based Experiential Assessment as a Guide and Companion to EFT Intervention

1. Attachment security—the key target of assessment and change—offers a benchmark and a beacon of hope and a pathway home.
2. Attachment informs our understanding of the potential impacts of trauma.
3. A developmental frame guides understanding, pacing, and intervention.
4. EFT is fundamentally a nonpathologizing approach.
5. The surface symptom picture can be at least partially understood as a manifestation of underlying attachment insecurity.
6. The focus is on present process.
7. The therapist tunes in and finds focus with CARE in initial sessions and maintains attention to these four dimensions throughout the therapy process.

8. Safety is established and maintained with attention to PACE.
9. Ongoing assessment guides intervention.
10. Client strengths and resources are illuminated.

PACE

Therapy is structured and safety is established at outset and maintained throughout the therapeutic process with careful attention to PACE:

Pacing the process with attention to capacity
Accurate and on-target reflections
Collaboration
Empathic attunement and therapist presence

6

Finding Focus and Maintaining Momentum in Stage 1

At the beginning of Session 8, Saul tells his therapist, "I am impressed about where we go in session. We hit deep veins. I'm intense and therapists just can't handle me. But you follow my line of thought. I'd had no access to deeper parts for years and now I have a path. But I still carry this weight of my despicableness. I am a traitor."

Indeed, Saul is intense. Fascinating, obviously brilliant, and very difficult to guide, to focus, and to interrupt as he launches into long discussions of his life, moving from philosophy to poetry to multiple labels for his problems. The rhythm of the first sessions was, generally, long, dense speeches from Saul, during which the therapist worked hard to find core themes and emotional elements and reflect them back to Saul, followed by Saul correcting the therapist with a "Yes, but . . . ," always adding complicated qualifications, rebuttals, and long digressions. The therapist was fascinated, challenged, and by the end of each session, likely exhausted.

Saul was referred as a "trauma survivor and war vet." The picture that emerged was that he suffered from symptoms of PTSD, such as intrusive thoughts and memories, and he certainly had experienced traumatic stress, but it helped the therapist more to see him as dealing with an emotional disorder characterized by anxiety, anger, and depression triggered by his family history, his injury at the end of his arduous training as an elite commando, and the chronic pain and surgeries that followed. He now lived on the other side of the world from his family on a farm in Canada with his wife, their infant daughter, and his dogs. In spite of constant pain from his back injury, conflicts with his partner, and inner turmoil, he had, in the two years before therapy, turned the farm into a model of innovative conservation-oriented productivity. What stood out about Saul from the very first session was the explicit contempt with which he described himself and the labels he offered as to who he was: *pathetic, selfish, weak, too much, traitor, ingrate, disgusting, despicable,* with *hideous* and *broken* prominent on this list. He noted that he spends his life trying to "escape" these judgments. The judgments arose mostly from his perception of this relationship with his family but also from his military service. He was injured right at the end of years of intense military training, noting with contempt in his voice, "I finished that commando course marching at the ceremony with my comrades, but I was LIMPING like a freak!"

It is significant that he also noted his longing to belong, since attachment theory tells us that shame is, in essence, about a sense of unworthiness, and therefore, a loss of hope of acceptance and secure belonging. It is part of the inner model of self ("I am unworthy and unlovable") and also about the sensitivity to and fear of being negatively evaluated by others ("Others will reject me") and most often triggers withdrawal from others. Saul described being in a "straightjacket" caught between wanting to belong and feeling unworthy and wanting to escape and be alone. Trauma is so often accompanied by shame and self-disgust, especially when the traumatic experience is delivered when we are young by the ones we are supposed to be able to count on and love. We blame ourselves rather than face the pain of how cruel and indifferent these attachment figures were. Nevertheless, the level and intensity of Saul's self-denigration was unique and was presented in a rational, intellectual tone as the incontrovertible truth.

The recurring pattern of affect regulation and engagement with others that began to take shape in the first sessions and are captured in Move 1 of the EFIT Tango was best described as a sense of being stressed and frustrated, free-flowing anger accompanied by tension and nausea, and a flood of judgments about himself. He would then shut down and turn away from interactions with others, often going off into the woods with his dogs, telling himself that alone was better, philosophizing about the nature of life, and feeling hopeless and depressed. This pattern would then recur, becoming self-sustaining and self-maintaining.

In terms of exceptions to being caught in this pattern, he noted that he used to write journals and poetry until a few years ago when he found that he just could not put pen to paper, but that he had recently begun to tentatively turn and try to talk to his partner, Netty, about his turmoil. He acknowledged that she was very caring and supportive, even though they still fought all the time. The therapist framed his strengths and resources as his three-year relationship with his partner, his commitment to his farm and love of the natural world, his intellect, his loving connection with his dogs, as well as his courage in dealing with his injuries and pain and coming to Canada to shape a new life. Reaching for a grounding metaphor, the therapist often referred to him as a warrior fighting a battle within himself and in his life.

To be able to focus the sessions, it soon became necessary for the therapist to explicitly name the cycle between Saul and the therapist, and reflect the process of the sessions. The therapist made the goals clear in terms of working to order his flow of experience and finding the most powerful emotional patterns that kept him in his straightjacket and his "depression." They put together the dance of the therapist's attempts to do this—to focus down on the heart of the matter—and his responses, mostly interruptions and qualifications, which took them off into another general intellectual level, talking "about" matters and offering information rather than delving deeper. The therapist then outlined the planned response to keep them focused so that he could move into a different place in his life. This involved telling him that the therapist would do their best to listen, and that his ideas and comments were often fascinating, however, the therapist would sometimes simply stop him by saying, "I am going to stop you. I want us to stay focused here." And then the therapist would ask him to return to the path they had been following and stay with them there. He consented to this. While doing this, the therapist would use a poignant image or statement from the present session or even from a moment in a past session to refocus him, repeating it in an evocative voice and slow pace. This was a bumpy ride at first but became easier and easier as Saul began to trust this new dance and allowed the therapist to direct the session. At these moments, the therapist was ever grateful for the EFIT map to Saul's inner world that allowed them to pinpoint where to go, and how to stay and explore the leading edge of his experience. The therapist remained aware of his sensitivity and his level of tolerance for actually staying in contact with this leading edge.

There is much more to say about this fascinating client. The following is an extensive transcript of the whole of Session 11, where the therapist was generally able to use the five moves of the EFIT Tango to keep the session focused and flowing.

THERAPIST: What I heard you saying last session was, "I decided I was impossible to love," and there was a lot from your brother with his complete apparent inability to relate to or respond to your pain, and also his kind of very narrow definition of what maleness should be, which was your model. But then you also talked about how you'd been seeking, longing for, you used the word "longing," seeking and longing for this connection with other men in your life. And you'd occasionally achieved it for a moment, it seemed, but then it would disappear. So, I thought that was really important, both the longing and the deciding that it must be that you're impossible to love. And we did talk, you said at the end, "When I really think about that, I feel grief, but I also know that I'm coping and doing things like mentoring other men and my volunteers. And I have my lady, Netty." But the other thing you said that was interesting, because I realized I hadn't asked you about it, was that you said, and I'm not sure about the timing of this, it was a bit confused in my notes. You said there was a big, first main depression. I think you talked about it happening when you were about 23 or 24, but I could be wrong.

SAUL: Yeah, yeah.

THERAPIST: And what really hit me about that was you said, "Basically in that depression, my self was obliterated." So those two things really hit me as incredibly important. And we've talked in other sessions about how emotionally alone you were, growing up, with you holding your mother's soul in your hand and having no safety in this connection. But longing for connection with your brother. Your father was very busy, absent. All this unfulfilled longing, this need to belong . . .

SAUL: And you know what's funny, I forgot to mention that, but even early on in life, I had this very strong longing, almost a desperation. I guess, maybe, I did feel deep down unfulfilled with my relationship with my brother. Even when I was growing up and we were close. And it's funny, it started even before the military. I guess it's always been in me, that sense of longing for, like, a brother or masculine connection that is nourishing, but I guess. . . . Yeah, even earlier than I realized, I didn't make that connection with depression, and always meeting disappointment there. And it's funny because romantically, like with women, I've had more success than most men.

THERAPIST: Yes. I have this image of you as this sensitive little boy. And you know, there are certain things that are common to all of us. You wanted, you longed for this sense of intimacy and connection. And what I hear is that, with your mother, that came at too high a price. She gave you nurturing on a certain level, but it came with an enormous set of price tags. You said you "had to carry her soul" and always be her little boy and protect her from her anxiety. And so, the natural thing for you, I think, was to look for a male figure to get that sense of safety and connection, and it just wasn't there.

SAUL: Well, the funny thing is that in all that longing, I never considered my father. That's quite funny because in all of this looking and just clinging to my brother or to my crew mates in the army or friends here or there, I've never turned to my father.

THERAPIST: Well, when you first talked about your father, I think way back in the first session, I got the very clear impression that you knew that he just wasn't available. He was distracted; he was busy; he was focused somewhere else. So, it was very natural that you turned to your older brother, right?

SAUL: I mean, when I was growing up, I knew that if I would go to my father, all I would get would be some kind of patriotic spiel about being strong or whatever. It's funny, because in all this longing for a father figure or for a brother, I never really even considered my father.

THERAPIST: Yes. So what interests me is the effect that this has had on the emotional patterns in your life. Okay?

SAUL: Yeah, I actually wanted to talk about that. In a way, it's funny you mentioned that. I wanted to. . . . Well, I wanted to be a bit more specific than that. I actually wanted to maybe talk and, you know, we haven't talked much about my relationship, my romantic relationship. But of course, yeah, in many ways my relationship with my mother, as well, has really shaped my relationship with women. I know that relationships, especially romantic relationships, I think, is your field of expertise or your focus of research.

THERAPIST: Yeah. And we can do that. [This becomes the focus in session 13.] I guess I just want to hang out here for a bit. [Refocus.] You help me, you help me fill in the blanks. If we just stay here with your longing for this connection with a man, however you see that, you know, you can see it when you're little as a father figure, or you can see it as a brother or a friend. When you think of that longing, you help me understand. If I look at the way it unfolds, in a general way, whether we're looking at you with your friend in school, your brother, the men that you talked about in your crew that were so important to you, that basically how it unfolds is that you have this deep longing for connection and intimacy, to be seen and responded to by a male figure. It's really active in you. You have this deep longing. And so, what you do, being you, with your intense aliveness, what you do is you reach, you try to show up emotionally. You might talk about your hurt. I think you tried to talk about your hurt with your brother and how this was just impossible to do. You might talk about vulnerability. You reach, you long, you reach. And sometimes . . . [Staying with the focus of isolation, longing and deprivation—deeper need and the pattern of interactions.]

SAUL: I also just try to come close, in general, to that person.

THERAPIST: Right? Okay. So, you reach, you try to get close, and then what happens with your brother or with your crew, sometimes you would get a little of this connection, this feeling of belonging. You'd get it. It would be there. But inevitably, somehow, you wouldn't be able to rely on it. It would sort of evaporate. The person would turn and move away.

SAUL: It would get too close. It would get too much for the person. It would get too intense for the person. It's not just that it would evaporate. It would end.

THERAPIST: Okay. It would get too intense.

SAUL: Too close. Especially for men. It's too close. Men are taught to, especially in masculine connections, are supposed to be more casual. Supposed to be more. . . . It's also what the people have had the courage to tell me. I know it was too much. It's just too much for them.

THERAPIST: But too much. I'm playing with "too much," okay? "Too much" is that this connection was too intense for them, over-whelming for them. So then, what they would do is they would turn away from you—disappoint you. So inevitably this has ended up with hurt and disappointment, yes? And then, you said last session, there is grief, real hurt and grief. And then, you help me, what would come up? You would try to understand this. And you would find yourself saying, which is so normal, because the first place we look is kind of inside us, "Well, it's me, it's me. I must be impossible to love. And there must be something basically, some-how, deficient about me or different or strange or unacceptable. It's me." And then, you help me, there would not only be grief, hurt, and disappointment, there would also be a kind of a despair that comes when we say to ourselves, "It's me. I will never find this closeness that I need. It's me. There's something somehow impos-sible or off about me." [Interpretation linking deprived longing to self-abnegation to despair.] Then usually, you tell me, we usually find that this is a black, clear road straight into depression, straight into despair. Because you know, "I'm never gonna get what I need, and it's me. There's something wrong with me. If I get close enough to be seen, I'm not loved and seen, I'm somehow always turned away from as too much. It's me." That has to leave you with a feel-ing of helplessness and despair. Or maybe you have a better word because you used the word for your depression, you used the word "self-obliterating." And I'm not quite sure how that resonates for you. But it leads you into depression. Then you struggle out of this darkness and you come back again. And the same thing happens again and again, yeah? Longing, reaching with so much need, and finding no one. Deciding you are unlovable—obliterates you—and you shut down and withdraw into depression, and there, even more hurt and longing waits for you so you try again to connect and find anger but also deeper despair. Yes? [Move 1 of the Tango—the inner and between process patterns that structure the symptom are outlined and made the problem.]

SAUL: Yeah. Maybe you're right. Maybe this is what is at the core of the matter. I mean, I have never personally interpreted these rejections as the main drive behind my despair or my depressions. But, you know, maybe it is, because in the end, when you feel like you belong. . . . It's more difficult to despair when you feel like you have a place in the world. But I've always, I've looked at many, many other traumas like what we have talked about, with me being very stunted and very sheltered, focused on keeping my mother happy and letting her swaddle me, and then kind of throwing myself into the military to be the opposite of that. I already had a very strong propensity for melancholy, which might have not culminated in a full-spectrum depression but was omnipresent growing up. And I mean, yeah, maybe . . . the thing is, rejection was something that I experienced long before I really understood how much I wanted this kind of connection. Even when I was still connected to my brother. I think maybe it's confusing because I sometimes have a tendency to caricaturize my brother. But I felt very connected to him, even though in hindsight, I realized that it was toxic for me and that he wasn't the right person to be able to see me. But growing up and until I was around 23 or 24, I was very, very close with him. When I was growing up, we would talk. We'd talk on the phone twice a day even when he was not living at home anymore. But on the other hand, there was a sense of rejection because he couldn't see all of me. But I didn't want to see all of myself either. But the rejection was more present in my social life in school. I didn't have friends. I became more and more self-conscious and acutely self-aware, my social prospects dwindled, and in the end, disappeared completely. I didn't have any friends and I felt very rejected by everyone. They called me a mamma's boy.

THERAPIST: Yeah, well, maybe rejection is just one piece of the pie. Maybe the other piece of the pie is not just rejection, but isolation and that feeling of not belonging, which also feeds into, "I'm different. There's something wrong with me. I don't belong. I'm not one of the boys. I don't have a place in the world." That whole feeling of, "Somehow it must be me," that is hard. Those things, that frustrated longing, that aloneness.

SAUL: Yeah, I'm sure. I think. . . . I agree that it's one of the major contributors. I think there are other ones and it's, you know, who can say? It's hard to rank things in order of magnitude or in level of influence on the soul. But I'm sure that was a huge part. But in another way, I'm also asking myself if this kind of isolation is not also the result of something . . . if it's not a symptom of something that's a lot more foundational. [The therapist feels a segue into intellectual, almost abstract reflection.] I have been and still am, very, very different from the men around me or the people around me. And when I look at the people that I grew up with and the life that, in the end, I chose, and how I live my life, it's quite objectively easy to say that I was very different, even when I was young. And I felt that I knew that. I felt that, even though I didn't know that I was going to end up this far from the world that I came from, I knew that I was very different. And, you know, the way for me to kind of rationalize that was that I said that I felt, because I was living in the United States until I was five, I would say, "Well, I feel more connected to the American culture or European culture than my own culture." That was a way for me to try to reject the vulgarity and the pushiness and the violence of his culture, and to try and. . . . But I felt different, so, you know, in a way, this rejection, this isolation, this longing, in a way, could be just a symptom or a manifestation of something that's more foundational.

THERAPIST: Well, I'm not sure if things are more or less foundational, but certainly what you're talking about fits here, because, you know, it's kind of like, we all want to belong. And what that means when we're little is lots of times, especially when we're in groups or when we have figures that we look up to, like an older brother, we want to know that we are like them. And there's kind of a sameness that's comforting. And what I'm hearing for you is that you always knew. You always knew. [Therapist redirects, regains focus on sense of belonging.]

SAUL: I think there was a tremendous frustration in me because, in the end, the gifts that I do have. . . . They were never accepted, and they were never acknowledged, let alone cherished. I had no respect for any of the teachers that I met in my 12 years in school, for example. A more poetic or philosophical propensity in me or things that are a bit more artistic, never . . . hmm. I was constantly pushed in directions that I didn't care for, and I could be good enough just by mustering force of will and applying myself. So, I was a pretty good basketball player. I'll tell you the truth: I hated it. I hated every second of it. I hated being in that team. I felt so self-aware. I was so afraid of getting the ball, of having the ball passed to me. You know, for example, I was very good at math and physics and sciences, but . . . school was easy for me. So none of my skills were ever . . .

THERAPIST: Let's slow down a minute.

SAUL: Developed.

THERAPIST: Because I want to go back to what you said. [Redirect from philosophical discussion.] The most basic thing you said was, "When I think about this pattern in my life, this pattern of longing, wanting to be close and trying to reach to be close, there is the wanting to be seen and accepted for who I was, wanting to be seen and accepted." Then finding that not only sometimes were you too intense, but you were just different. You weren't what people expected from a male child in that culture, right? So, you know, that brings grief and even more longing. And that brings, you know, just a feeling of somehow never being accepted, never being let in, and that's the place where you say, "I'm impossible to love." And you go into despair and grief and helplessness, and to where you feel obliterated. That feeling that you have, of your gifts, yourself, not being seen and accepted. I mean, that is kind of like the core of most people's pain that they experienced as a child. [Move 3—deepening engagement with core emotion: desperate longing and shame, but still on a discursive level.]

SAUL: What I'm trying to emphasize is that it wasn't just that I didn't feel seen with others. You know, some people can be very isolated, but they can find a gift or a skill that gives them a sense of fulfillment and sense of self.

THERAPIST: Yes, I hear you. But you never found that. You tried to do what was expected of you.

SAUL: So, what I'm saying is that it wasn't just that belonging. It was also, I think, a frustration of a soul that isn't finding ways to express itself. And that becomes self-destructive, when a mind or a soul doesn't have ways to express their gifts. And sometimes they just turn to destroying things on the inside. And so, I guess, the isolation, yes, it's an important part. But I also think that one of the things that was the hardest for me is that I didn't have anything of my own that I felt was of value. There was no skill that I took pride in. You know? Yes, I was a really good student, but I didn't care about that. I didn't care about it enough to even go to school. I would just study a bit for an exam. And yes, I was on the basketball team. I didn't care about that either. There was nothing I had that I cared about. [Saul's philosophizing is where he feels confident and competent but also disconnects him/distances him from his experience—protection becomes prison.]

THERAPIST: Yeah. That is a key part of how we decide when we're growing up and when we're little, how valuable we are, because we have certain ways of being or talents that others say, "Oh, that's good. That's great." And we somehow feel, "Ah, not only am I belonging, but I'm of value here." What I'm hearing is you didn't get that. You had to accommodate your mum and her anxiety and need to protect you, along with your brother's image of a macho Saul. So, we're putting together all these feelings that go on under this depression. But I'm still somehow hung up here, perhaps because of our first few sessions where you talked to me so much about the fact that when you got caught in these down feelings, whatever we call them, that you'd get lost in . . . let's use one word that you used, you used "self-disgust." You'd get caught in self-disgust. So, this seems to be a core part of this problem. When we are not seen and accepted by others at all, when we don't get the feeling that who we are, our special self, is valuable and belongs and can be related to, we doubt our own value. We feel alien, somehow, and that leads straight into the sort of self-disgust you're talking about, straight into what I picked up from the last session, which is, "I'm impossible to love." Right? [Saul used to block this frame previously, saying it was "heresy"—against the family code that said that he was a traitor, that he was the problem.]

SAUL: The self-disgust. I feel like there's a very strong interwoven piece there of my mother and how that relationship was perceived by my peers and my brother. The self-disgust comes, I think, very much from a sense of being reliant or dependent or weak, and then resenting that and so, somehow being selfish or ungrateful. Somehow spoiled. Somehow spoiled.

THERAPIST: Needy. Reliant.

SAUL: That's when I feel disgusted.

THERAPIST: Yeah. Remember we talked about how, of course as a human being, you're dependent, of course you are. Of course, you need someone to rely on. And the only one around most of the time was your mother. And the deal with your mother, the price, was that you carry her soul, which was, it's like, suffocating? Never to upset her was the rule. But being with her is the only show in town. It's the only place you can get this nurturance. So of course, you go there because you have to in order to survive. I get that. But I want to know, if we just stay with that phrase.

SAUL: "Self obliteration" or . . . ?

THERAPIST: Well, we've talked about lots of key things. (*Therapist slows down, soft voice.*) Loneliness, isolation, you know, never feeling valued, never feeling seen. We've talked about longing, hurt, sadness. And yes, all these things obliterate our sense of a valid, concrete, valued self—all these things. But I want to know, if we just focus on one phrase, if we just focus down on times when you would get to the place where you'd say to yourself, "Well, I'm not seen. I'm not the way I should be. I'm not valued. I'm not like these other people. I'm different. And therefore, I'm impossible to love." I want to know, when you let that sit for a minute, what is triggered by all this not belonging and isolation and differentness? When you let that sit for a moment, what happens for you? What do you feel in your body? [Affect assembly.]

SAUL: I feel kind of lethargic. It makes me feel despondent. And when I think back to how I felt growing up or how I felt with my crewmates or other times like this, I just want to crumple. We talked about that, wanting to sag, kind of collapse around my chest, but also a sense of lethargy. That is very much the defining characteristic of my depressions—an inability to muster anything for any reason.

THERAPIST: There's kind of a shutdown of your energy. There's no life energy coming. The feeling in your body is, "I just want to crumble. I just want to sag. I just want to collapse." [Specifying the label "depression" as experienced.]

SAUL: Yeah, no life energy is a very good way to put it. I feel severed from the wellspring of life in that kind of moment. Yeah, I feel severed from instinct or body or soul or anything.

THERAPIST: You're kind of lost here? You're sort of lost in space. You just want to crumble. Yeah. I got it.

SAUL: I guess crumple, crumple.

THERAPIST: All right, crumple. So, here's the trigger. You have this longing. You so want this contact. You so want to be seen. You so want to know that the essence of who you are is precious and valuable. You so want to know that someone can see you, not as different or strange or not acceptable, but as just Saul and that you're accepted and you are allowed to come close. And you so want these things. And suddenly, when you are rejected, when you get the opposite message, your body goes into no energy, you know, lost in space. Crumpling. [Emotional handle—door to deeper inner reality.]

SAUL: But the thing that I find the most curious is that now that I do have that in my life, well, I do have someone who believes in me and sees me and knows that I'm different, but thinks that it's wonderful, and I can't take that in. And in many ways, I feel like rejecting her for that. [Client shifts the level of experiencing, disengages from specific inner experience.]

THERAPIST: Of course. For years and years and years this has been your experience. The dreadful irony for most of us is that our brain says, "This is the way it goes." Our nervous system says, "Here we go. This is the dance. This is the way it goes. I know it's gonna go this way." So then ironically, when we've experienced something for years, in order to have some sort of sense of control over it, we predict it. And then someone comes along who doesn't do what we expect and who answers our longing. And yes, you've just said something very profound. We don't quite know how to take that in, how to trust that, because we're still caught in a sense of rejection and the possibility of crumpling. We're still caught in carefulness, right? So we don't quite know what to do when things change. But I want to know . . . [Therapist validates his block to taking in this frame and attempts to redirect.]

SAUL: It's worse than that. It's not just not knowing how, it's almost like something in me feels, there's almost, like a derision toward that person that is like this. There must be something wrong with them.

THERAPIST: Well of course, because if we go back to, "I'm impossible to love," if somebody turns and says, "No, you're my special one and I love you," some part of your brain says, "You're a fool. You're an idiot." [Therapist highlights how model of self impacts/blocks ability to take in love and care.]

SAUL: Yeah. Yeah.

THERAPIST: Right? [Redirect back into direct experience accessed above—affect assembly.] I want to stay with this, this feeling of differentness, isolation, and your body goes into lethargy. It's lost in space. But I want to know what happens. What do you say to yourself in those moments? Like we've come up with, "I'm impossible to love." But what do you say to yourself when crumpling? Is that the main thing you say, "This longing is there but . . . I'll never be loved?"

SAUL: No, I don't think about that. I don't think about being loved.

THERAPIST: What comes up for you when you feel these feelings? Can you feel them now? Can you feel what this feeling of wanting to crumple feels like?

SAUL: Yeah, yeah.

THERAPIST: Okay. All right. So if you stay with this . . .

SAUL: What I say. I kind of more levitate toward a kind of existential crisis or existential despair, where I say, "Well, what's the point of it? You know, life isn't worth it anyhow." Or, "There's no point in even trying," or, "I don't care enough to try and I don't care if I live or die," and, "I don't care about anything." I just go to a place of numbness and indifference. And I usually just try to find a way to numb myself.

THERAPIST: Ah. Despair. No point.

SAUL: I don't do drugs or drink or anything, but I did use video games for many years to hide from myself and numb myself. And I do start excessive eating or excessive sleeping. But I never think about, "Oh, I can't be loved."

THERAPIST: Okay, so let's stay there a minute, because what you just said is so important. You said, "Okay, we know what the triggers are here. We've talked about them, and then my body starts to crumple, crumple, and all the energy leaves me." Right? And when you say to yourself, "I'm impossible to love," that is kind of a meta thing. But what you say to yourself in the moment is, "There's no point. There's no point. Don't try. It doesn't matter if I live or die. What does it matter? I don't care." Right? And then what comes along with that is a numbness.

SAUL: I don't know. Yeah. The numbness, I think, is just my way to try and shut that out.

THERAPIST: Yeah, I hear you. And what you used to do in that numbness, is you used to distract yourself with video games or with food or with lots of sleep. And you help me, is that a picture of Saul's basic depression? Is that the basic animal? Is that the depression that just used to obliterate you? Because, of course, that numbness, that feeling of, "I don't care anyway. The only way I can survive is not to care," that is, in a way, self-obliteration. It's like you just kind of give up on being a self, right?

SAUL: Yeah, but it's beyond a simple kind of reorganization. So, it's not just that I will quit my studies and quit my job and move back to my parents' house and just live in my childhood room like an animal in a cage. It goes beyond these kinds of external reorganizations. Sometimes when I truly go to a very dark place, like I have in the last three years, where with the disability and pain where I was bedridden and the enormous onset of trauma that has been resurfacing in relationship to my family life, it's an obliteration. I call it an obliteration of the self, because I've experienced that enough times to know. . . . When I come out from that, if I come out from that, it's almost like being a different person. This last depression completely reorganized my soul, my personality, and my belief systems, to quite a substantial extent. [He exits from the focus on pain to make positive points.]

THERAPIST: Perhaps that's something wonderful and magical, isn't it? If you can go into these dark, dark places that you are talking about, where you say that there's no point, you feel this sense of crumple. You say, "I'll never belong." Right? "I'm not like other people." You crumple. "There's no point." Right? "So, I'm not gonna try. There's no point in trying, just give up." And you go numb, and you go into just, somehow trying to find ways to distract yourself, right? And then . . . [Reflect, recap, repeat emotional handles to deepen experience—Move 2 of the Tango.]

SAUL: Almost like a cocoon. It's almost a cocoon.

THERAPIST: That's good.

SAUL: Larva emerges from a cocoon as a different thing.

THERAPIST: That's a beautiful image. And what you're saying is somehow in this obliteration of self, this cocoon you go into, you manage, you do manage to come out and renew yourself and learn from that experience. That's an incredible strength, isn't it, Saul? [Accept and validate his positive frame/strength—this is also an exit from painful experience.]

SAUL: Well, there's also something deeply tragic about it. I sometimes lose things that are so sacred to me, things that I could not imagine life without, and I can lose them to an extent that I can never find them again. And that makes me question the very existence of something sacred in this life or the very existence of something that is.

THERAPIST: So, let's talk about . . . [Therapist wanting to go back to the specific and concrete emotional level.]

SAUL: And even the existence of a love that can overcome. And I've lost some things—I used to write.

THERAPIST: Tell me.

SAUL: I used to write a lot, and I used to feel like there is nothing that could ever change my dedication to that, and nothing that could sway me from that. But now I can't write. It makes me nauseous to think about writing. Makes me want to throw up, to think about reading anything that I wrote. I feel sickened by it. So, you know, yes, there is. I think that in many ways I've had to undergo truly being reborn. But also, it's exhausting to have to learn how to live the most basic aspects again. Now I'm in the process of trying to learn how to live again, having been bedridden for three years and in deep depression, and then in complete disability and despair, and you know, I'm trying to learn how to be human again, how to exist again. And I do know that in the end, that will make me profound. But it also . . . I'm so tired.

THERAPIST: Hey, Saul.

SAUL: I'm so tired.

THERAPIST: Hey, Saul.

SAUL: Mm-hmm.

THERAPIST: I hear you. That's so tiring. And we lose things along the way, right? But my sense is that for many, many people, maybe yours has been more intense, but for many, many people that is the journey of life. You have to go through the darkness, and you have to reinvent yourself. [Normalizing and saying that this is human and he belongs.] But you're saying, "Here I am again, learning how to be human," but from my view out here, I want to say, "Hey, Saul, that's hard and exhausting, and you lose things along the way. But you're doing pretty well, aren't you?" [Resource; validate strengths.]

SAUL: I don't know that I am. I mean, I still can't find. . . . To me, there's nothing. . . . I can have so much in this world, like externally, but if I don't feel like . . . there's no temple mount. I don't feel like I carry something that is sacred inside of me. Like I don't have a connection to the profound, the more philosophical or poetic.

THERAPIST: Well . . . [Change of level again. Does the therapist follow or try to go back?]

SAUL: You know, life can feel meaningless to me. That's what I struggle with day to day.

THERAPIST: Yes, yes, but . . . (Saul interrupts.)

SAUL: I have so much to be grateful for. I have a beautiful daughter, a beautiful partner. I'm working toward fulfilling my dreams of healing forests, and, you know, yeah. But I feel more empty inside than I did when I was living alone in an attic, writing and meditating and running with my dog. And I felt so full back then. And I feel so empty so much of the time now.

THERAPIST: Well, we'll go into that, okay? We'll talk about that, all right? But right now, I want you to look at the things that you've said, which is that you do come out of that dark place, and some-times you've lost things, like your ability to write. You can't do that anymore. And I thought it was particularly interesting when you talked about that you don't want anyone to read what you've writ-ten, which is a bit like you don't want to be seen, right? You don't want to put yourself up for that kind of possible rejection. And you have lost a lot in all these struggles. [Therapist reflects but also tries to return to main themes of the session.]

SAUL: I did want people to read what I wrote before. I mean, when I used to write, I wanted people to read it. It's only now that I can't read it or see it.

THERAPIST: Right. But basically, you've had to learn, again and again, to be human, right? And what you're telling me is, "And in all this, I still struggle with a feeling of, somehow, what is the meaning of this? What is the meaning of life? Is there something sacred?" And also, you tell me that maybe you are not sure what the temple mount is, but that you have meaning in being a father, in being a partner, in healing the forest, in planting your trees. [Accepts client's frame and emphasizes the strengths as well.]

SAUL: What I'm saying is I don't doubt that there is meaning in life and that there is meaning in what I do. There is something sacred in life. What truly hurts me is that I don't feel like I can touch it. I don't feel like I can feel it. I know I'm surrounded by it. I know I bring something to the people around me, to my family, even to the for-est, something sacred to them, but I can't feel that in myself. I can't feel. . . . In myself, I feel severed. I feel like I'm severed from some kind of deep wellspring in myself. And I try to meditate, go into a sense of flow, to accept life for all its complexity and tragedy.

THERAPIST: My goodness, Saul, what's coming up for me . . . is I just want you to notice . . . your mother put a weight on you when you were a child to "carry her soul," be her baby boy so she could handle her anxiety. And now, you put so much weight on you here. You're telling me you've been through three years of pain and dis-ability, touching all your pain from childhood and a sense of not being the superman commando—the one that saves the nation. You're saying, "I've had to reinvent myself again and again, walk through pain and darkness to the point where everything seemed pointless . . . my very self was obliterated. Depression, helplessness, emptiness, and pain. And I am doing good things in my life. But somehow, somehow, I can see that things I'm doing are sacred. But I can't quite, can't, can't own that, touch it, take it in." Is that right? [Reflect, repeat emotional themes—handles.]

SAUL: Okay. Yeah. Yeah.

THERAPIST: Hmm. I hear, "I can't quite be my ideal poetic and philosophical and artistic self, I am limping still, as I did when I came down from the mountain with my army crew." My response is, "Right," because you've been caught in this pattern that we were talking about. You've been caught up in this emotional dance and let's just take one part of the dance. If you're numbing out, if you're numbing out and hunkering down and trying to shut everything down just to deal with all this pain, you better believe that your emotions somehow become vaguer and vaguer. They're like a music you can't even hear. And you better believe that then you end up feeling empty. Right? And sometimes it takes time to hear, listen, and trust yourself again. [Move 5 of the Tango—Integration but also setting up emotional engagement for a possible Move 3.] I want you to notice all the important things you've said in this session so far about the feelings that you get caught in, the crumple in your body. How you tell yourself, "There is no point." You hunker down and then you struggle and have found ways to burst out of that cocoon, to come to life. And this is a struggle—it is exhausting, and you feel a sense of loss. This is Saul's life. I want to know, if you look at little Saul, I think way back, we talked about little Saul at around 11 years old, when you first began to feel the real "stings of rejection" from your classmates.

SAUL: I didn't feel like that at all when I was real small, growing up. That was like the golden time, the golden era of our family. I felt very loved and very cherished, and pretty much until I was five.

THERAPIST: Right. And then somehow, that picture all changed. (*Using soft, slow prosody.*) The beginnings of this dance, this dark dance, this dance of depression, started up, the beginnings of aloneness and rejection from your brother, the music of, "I must be impossible to love. There's no point. This is somehow terribly sad. I've got all this longing. It doesn't go anywhere." Yes? (*He nods.*) The beginnings of all that started up, and little Saul said, "There must be something wrong with me. There's no point. I'm just not what people want and to be what my mother wants, I have to disappear—never feel. I will be the warrior my brother demands but I can never limp! I don't belong. I'm impossible to love. I must be despicable." When you think of little Saul, of course he couldn't verbalize all those things. But when you think of little Saul, I want you to actually close your eyes and see him, if you can. [Move 3.] Maybe see him standing in a place—his room or somewhere in nature where he would go—and you can see little Saul. You can see his face. You can see what clothes he has on. You look at him and you are aware of the beginnings of all this, all this exhausting turmoil and longing and pain that is beginning in him. And you see how he longs to be seen and how he doesn't belong. I want you to try to see him. I want you to let yourself feel the way he feels. What would you say to him? Well, first of all, can you see him? Can you see him?

SAUL: I see something. I can see him at a certain point. I can see myself with a certain kind of longing. And I dunno, there's a point where, I don't know why, I remember some evening that I was standing in front of the mirror after a shower or something. For some reason it got blazed into my mind. [This is new. Previously he would say "No, I can't see him," or "I don't want to look." Window of tolerance/capacity is widening but is still small.]

THERAPIST: All right, so when you see this, what happens in you? What comes up for you? [Move 2 of the Tango—evocative question.]

SAUL: I just feel I am. . . . Well, what came to me, actually, was a very strong memory of myself standing in front of the mirror and thinking about this girl that I was, well, desperately in love with and I wanted more than anything, but realizing how absolutely hopeless it was, and how she would never have looked at me. I was so lost and quite troubled, and my self-esteem was not there. But I don't know. I just feel a deep, deep sadness for this boy that never had a chance to experience what people experience, to experience life.

THERAPIST: Right. To feel safe and accepted. To know he was precious.

SAUL: To participate in life. Never found a way to participate in life. Never found a place, never found . . . yeah. It's a grief, I guess it's a grief. [His face changes—he engages this emotion.]

THERAPIST: (Softly.) I want you to stay with this for a moment. How lost he was and how, you know, he wasn't really alive. He was just lost in all these feelings, right? And you feel this deep sadness for him. So, what would you like to do when you feel that sadness? Would you like to reach out and touch him? Would you like to say something to him?

SAUL: No, I would've just liked for him to see that one day he will come to lose respect for these things, for these people that he longed for, whose love he longed for so desperately, and that one day he will find a way to live a life that is a lot more integral than they could ever dream of. And that . . . [Shift to more intellectual level where he is comfortable. His window of tolerance for overwhelming emotion is still small.]

THERAPIST: Okay, so let's just stay there. So you would close your eyes, and you would say to him. . . . (*He doesn't close his eyes.*) I'd like you to close your eyes and see yourself doing that. Okay? You'd say to him, "There's a way through." [Returning to image but titrating risk of contact with vulnerable self so also focuses on the positive—there is a way out.]

SAUL: Well, I would say to him, "You're gonna go through hell, and this life is going to be very bitter. But there are moments of exquisite beauty. And that all of that pain and all that loss is what will lead you to a truer path."

THERAPIST: So, you would say to him, "There is a path, it's okay. There is a path. There is a path."

SAUL: It just goes through an abyss.

THERAPIST: Yeah. You help me. I think, on a very simple level, you might also say to him, "I see you. I see you. I see how lost you are. I see how hard it is for you. I see that you have all this longing, and you are desperately longing for love and it's not there. And it feels like it's never gonna be there." [Therapist distills core attachment pain—tries to deepen experience—keep the encounter going.]

SAUL: I don't know that I would've said that, just because knowing that little boy, he would not have wanted to hear that. Love was not. . . . What he really wanted more than anything was to have a place, was to feel like he was alive and to feel like he had a place. To be loved, yes, that's another something. But I don't think that he would've liked to hear that. [Therapist is aware that we are now at 60 minutes in a 75-minute session.]

THERAPIST: So, you'd like to say to him, "There is a path. You will have a place. You'll make a place. You will have a place."

SAUL: What I would say to him is, that, "There is no place, and there is no one, but you will go through loss and grief and pain, and you're gonna make a place for yourself."

THERAPIST: Ah, "You can make a place. You can find . . . "

SAUL: I would say to him, basically, what I would really want to say to him is, "There is no one, there is not going to be anyone along the path who is going to give you what you want. There is no one who is going to see you. There is no one who's going to offer you anything, any guidance, any meaning."

THERAPIST: Right, so you might say to him, "You're right. You are so alone right now. You are so lost right now. But you will make a place, you'll make a place."

SAUL: What I would say to him is, that, "You are right. You are different and you are going to feel very alone in this life. And that is the cross you're gonna have to bear. You're going to have to find the answers yourself."

THERAPIST: Goodness me. This is an awful lot to say to a little kid.

SAUL: Yeah, I guess, yeah. (*Laughs.*)

THERAPIST: But what I've heard you say is, "I would tell him, what I see when I look at you is I see how lost you are and what I wanna tell you is, yes, you are different. Yes, there's all these feelings of sadness and despair, but there is a path. And you will make a place. You will make a place." [Therapist tries to say with the simple and emotional, bypassing more philosophical levels.]

SAUL: I wasn't really a little kid. By the time I was 13, I was like a wizened old man, like just, there was something almost geriatric about me by then, I couldn't relate to children my age, you know. In a way, you know, I wasn't really a little kid by the time I was 11 or 12. I was already experiencing existential crises, full-blown ones. And yeah, I dunno.

THERAPIST: Right, right. It's true, isn't it, Saul? In spite of all these exhausting excursions into the dark, and in spite of all the pain and sorrow and loss, you have made a place for yourself. You are making a place for yourself.

SAUL: It's not in spite. It's not in spite of. It's because of. . . .

THERAPIST: Yes. Your pain has helped you grow. And in that place, like you said to yourself, there wasn't somebody who could answer your longing until you found a path and a place for you. You were alone. And indeed, you are finding a path and a place, and you have found a person who sees you and accepts you, even though that's hard for you to take in sometimes. You have said that when she comes close to you, you feel angry. Yeah? [Therapist reflects that Saul was close only with his mother who demanded his soul so that he had to shut down himself and his feelings. So, closeness is a threat—brings ambivalence. The dilemma of so many trauma survivors can be distilled as "closeness is impossibly dangerous and so is isolation and aloneness." The only solution is often to numb out and deny attachment longings. This dilemma is made explicit and worked on in future sessions in reference to his relationship with his partner.]

SAUL: Yes, but she can only see me and accept me because when I met her, I was strong, not in pain and disabled. There was something like the poetry and the philosophy and just the quality of soul that I had cultivated in me. So, it's not like she came and saw me in my despair and, you know, lifted me.

THERAPIST: Yeah, that is also what happens to us when we fall in love. Our self becomes more vital. Maybe you met her when you were on a high—just arrived in Canada. But since then, from what you've told me of your relationship, she's also seen you very, very low indeed. And she's still here.

SAUL: Yes. She is nurturing.

THERAPIST: Right. [Therapist accepts that this is Saul's limit in terms of deeper engagement with his pain for now.] So, what's it like to talk about all this? We've talked about a lot of stuff here. We've talked about the roots of your depression and your basic sort of emotional dance in life. How you blamed yourself for others not accepting you. What's it like to talk about this? [Move 4—Processing the Encounter.]

SAUL: I guess in a way, I feel, feel a kind of sense of resignation and like, realizing that the truth is that it has been like this from the beginning. That's what I would've liked to say to my young self.

THERAPIST: It's been like this. . . . It's been like this struggle, this battle, this having to reinvent yourself?

SAUL: Precisely. I've always been different, an outsider. Others have very, very rarely been able to be something that I need. For me.

THERAPIST: Yes, I get that.

SAUL: I don't know, I guess, how do I feel? One thing that you said and that really stuck with me is that you were talking about how you're not surprised that I don't feel a strong sense of vitality because I've been through so much in the last few years. And I guess what's hard for me is to remember that and to stay and to be patient.

THERAPIST: Yeah.

SAUL: Because I long, more than anything, I long for a connection to the profound, a connection to the deeper aspects of the self, to find a path back inward. And I guess it's hard for me to be patient because it feels like it's already been a lifetime of being bereft of something that is essential. But I guess when you talk about how these years have been quite difficult, I think that it's only been two years since my surgery. So, I guess, in that way, I have to. . . . Because deep down, I do know that healing is a process that you can't force—happens in deeper reaches of us.

THERAPIST: That's right.

SAUL: But it's hard for me to be patient sometimes, and I want it now. I want to feel more alive now.

THERAPIST: Well, you have a fierce and intense appetite for life. And you can also put those things into words, which lots of people can't, you know, that longing for the profound. People talk about it in different ways, but I think it is part of our human nature, that longing for what is deeper, what is, you know, what is the meaning of all this dance that we're caught in as human beings. Yeah, and it's hard to be patient. [Validate.]

SAUL: I think that once you've tasted it, once you've really, once you feel like you've really touched the sky, or when you feel like you've really touched something sacred, experienced life in a way that is much more colorful and vital than the everyday, your gonna want to feel that high again.

THERAPIST: Right, right. And I hear that, but I asked you what's it like to talk about this. And you said, "Well, what comes up is resignation because I realize I was always an outsider. I was always different. I wasn't gonna get what I needed. And then what comes up is this longing, this longing for the intense, the inner, the sacred, the profound part of life. And this longing, just like, is there, just, I longed for closeness and connection as a child. This longing comes up in me here." I guess I want to know, and I know that we need to end soon, but I want to know, when you think back to the little kid, do you also feel any tenderness for him? [Therapist asks because compassionate tenderness for vulnerable self is the antidote to shame and self criticism.]

SAUL: Not so much. No. No, I wouldn't say so.

THERAPIST: What do you feel for him?

SAUL: Maybe you could call it pity.

THERAPIST: All right.

SAUL: Like, I pity him for what he carries inside. I talked to you once about how being a boy, I used to lie in bed sometimes when I was trying to fall asleep. And I would close my eyes, and I would see inside of myself, a gulf of darkness, just an endless, bottomless abyss. And I could not illuminate it. I guess, sometimes I wonder how he's even alive, I guess. Yeah.

THERAPIST: It's almost like. . . . I have this image of you being able to say to him, "I see you and I see how hard life is and is going to be for you. And I'm sorry for it. And I feel pity for that." Yeah. [Therapist models the drama in proxy voice that Saul is unable to stay and shape. This is the least risky way to slide into Move 3.]

SAUL: I don't feel like there's anything I can really say to him that would help. In the end, he had to undergo these repeated deaths of his personality to try and develop any kind of sense of humanity.

THERAPIST: Yeah, and he found a path, which many people don't. And he made a place for himself. But I hear you. I'd like you to hold onto that pity. You said, "I don't think I can say anything." I'm not sure about that. I think this is about right now—that little child is still with you. Can you hear yourself saying to him, "I feel for you. I see you. I feel for you. I pity you. I see how hard it is for you. I see how intense your longing is to belong, to connect, to have people respond to you so you can have the real feeling of being alive and connected to deeper things. I see that. There's another place for you." Another place where he can have something that is his, something that he takes pride in. Something that is his, not just his dog. [Therapist reflects pride in self and life; is also an antidote to shame—builds secure sense of self.]

SAUL: But I can't say that I can feel compassion toward him. I don't know why.

THERAPIST: Well, pity's a kind of compassion, feeling sad for someone.

SAUL: Well, what I also feel like, well, often when I see someone in pain or . . . having experienced life the way I have, I don't see it as the kind of negative that needs to be abolished. I look at that boy and I think, "Well, he had to undergo what he underwent."

THERAPIST: So, you have covered a lot of ground today. A lot of ground. What I will try to do is sum it up. [Move 5 of Tango, Integrating and Validating, but we are overtime.] I'd also like you to think about the session after we are done because you did so much great work. I'd like you to sort of let it sit with you and let it hum for you, and sort of see what comes out of it, okay?

SAUL: Well, strange thing is that I say so much, it's almost like the moment I say it, it's gone. It's not easy for me to access.

THERAPIST: That's okay. You'll hang on to the bits that matter. Your nervous system will say, "This matters," and you will hold onto it. But I'll try to help you there, too. So, let's stop, and I'll try to see if I can write down a few key things and send to you. We'll meet next week, okay? And please take care of you.

Therapist summarizes five key points after the session and sends them to Saul. She also suggests that he now attempt to write down his memory of the session, in spite of his previous inability to write. He does, in fact, do this before the next session.

DISCUSSION OF THE SESSION

The transcript above is intended to show a Stage 1 session with a highly intellectual client being able to stay emotionally engaged and begin moving into a meaningful Move 3 emotional epiphany, or you could call it an *identity drama*. Saul begins to contact and accept his more vulnerable self—a self soundly rejected by his family. It is also an example of working with an intense and challenging client in EFIT. The therapist has to work hard to find and keep focus in the session and to encourage emotional engagement. Persistence and the repetition of the client's emotional handles are key. The EFIT map grounds the therapist and fosters the creation of this focus.

Saul's case is also interesting in that he was referred as a PTSD client, and although he did not do the usual PTSD measure (Trauma Symptom Inventory-2, TSI-2; Briere, 2011) so it is unknown how he might have scored on a formal test, he presented more explicitly with depression and an identity shaped by shame and self-denigration rather than a classical case of PTSD. His presentation fits with the EFIT formulation of PTSD as an emotional disorder, sharing classic core features with depression and anxiety disorders as laid out in the book *Attachment Theory in Practice* (Johnson, 2019). These features are: a chaotic stream of emotion that is deemed unacceptable; avoidance of pain and emotional issues, in Saul's case by staying with sophisticated intellectualizations; vigilance for cues of meaninglessness, pain, and shame; and a negatively skewed sense of self that cannot be revised from his intellectualized level of processing. As Damascio (1999) states, "Embodied experience is the ground that the self is created from."

Saul's version of the ever-recurring trauma trap that EFTers talk about is this: He stays distant from direct experience that might offer corrective experiences, valuing insight and philosophizing. He longs for connection but feels different, disgusting, and unlovable. He is sad but avoids this emotion. He then goes into a lethargy, a numbing cocoon where he does not feel alive but is caught in despair and loss. He cannot take in caring from his partner, almost despising her for her love. He pushes her away and feels ashamed, reminding himself that he is a traitor to his family and his military ideals. He then feels more disgusting and numbs more and finds life more and more meaningless while any sense of competent and worthy self is obliterated. This circular self-reinforcing pattern—his way of dealing with his trauma and pain—structures his daily life, his emotional reality, his relationships, and his identity. He explicitly names existential crises and indeed, helplessness brings up the core existential issues of isolation and not meaning much to others, choice in an uncertain universe—and the lurking pointlessness of life, meaning making—Saul wants to connect with the sacred, something bigger than himself, and the transient nature of life. He wants to "reinvent" himself and learn to feel human again. Our experience is that most trauma survivors long for this, not simply symptom management, as do most folks with any kind of emotional distress.

His present relationship with his partner seems typical of clients who have experienced significant injury in their attachment with their family of origin in that he longed for connection and also seemed threatened by it, and so often pushed his partner away. It is also hard for him, given his history, to trust and take in her caring when it is offered, which heightens his isolation. His trauma around being injured and finding himself disabled and in pain was addressed in therapy but he was already coping much better with this before therapy began, except for the shame element of being wounded, rather than heroically always resilient. We also addressed the cultural element of this, namely that his squad was seen and honored as the heroes and saviors of the nation and so viewed in an almost mythical light.

In terms of intervention, it was necessary to meet Saul where he was, so indeed the therapist joined him at the level of his intellect while going to the leading edge of his experience and attempting to open the door to his emotional realities. He was more open about his emotions in this session than previously but was still only able to touch his most vulnerable self for a short time. Some clients process their reality on a more cognitive level but can still learn to access and move through their emotions and so reach the moment where self and the dance of emotion are restructured.

Saul was a challenging client to keep focused and direct—to follow and to lead—but together, a place was reached where he was more securely connected with a competent worthy sense of self and with supportive others. A secure connection with self renders us strong and resilient—able to battle with the demons of trauma and to win.

FOLLOW-UP AFTER SESSION 11

Saul talks in Session 12 about how his perception of himself is improving but as this was celebrated and elaborated on, he discovered a contrasting sense of "pressure" in his temples and his chest. The thoughts that go along with this contrasting pressure are all about a sense of inadequacy: He thinks, "No. Really, I know that I am not enough," and then feels "exhausted." This makes sense. When our usual long-accepted sense of self is challenged, even in a positive way, this is stressful—new. The default is to go back to what we have always known. The conflict between new and old identity is exhausting, but more problematic is the letting go of the promise of the new sense of self.

The therapist explores this thought and his feeling of exhaustion with him, asking him who taught him to judge himself and when did he start doing this. He immediately remembered that his father and brother would tell him, beginning when he was around 8, that he was selfish and spoiled. His father was absent due to his high-level job, and his brother had moved out, so Saul lived with his highly anxious mother, who was totally focused on obsessively mothering him. The family law was that he was on no account to upset her by saying the wrong thing or talking about his feelings and worries. He says his temples hurt when he talks about this. He paints the picture of being alone with no friends and having to be her "little boy." If he upset her, he felt shame and would be criticized by his brother, so he shut down and spaced out, playing on his computer all the time. Finally, he rebelled and went from being his mother's little boy to working to join the most elite force of commandos, following in his father's footsteps and proving, as he saw it, that he was not "weak." This transition represented quite a leap.

The therapist expands on the sense of pressure in his head, and they come up with an image of a little boy in a terrible bind. He is alone and longing for love, but love is a dangerous place where you either have to betray or lose your sense of self or betray and wound the one you depend on and are supposed to protect. Either way you "commit treason" and are "a traitor"; these are some of Saul's favorite words. He related this dilemma to his present conflicts with his partner in which this pressure arises and he feels cornered and begins to get angry and has to escape. He also related this childhood bind to a recent incident when he was visiting his family and was called "spoiled, weak, and ungrateful" by his brother, and became so angry that he smashed his hand down and broke bones before fleeing from the family holiday completely. The therapist validates the fact that he allowed himself to protest and rage against his brother's accusations.

Bowlby points out in his writings that we do to ourselves as we have been done to. Saul pressures, doubts, and judges himself constantly. In this session, he is more and more emotionally engaged, moving into some level of a Stage 2 process, and the therapist attempts to set up a Move 3 encounter. First, the therapist tentatively explores beginning to share this pressure and shame with his mental image of his partner and then his image of his mother, but he does not engage with either of these. Returning to the image of him as a child caught in this bind of shame and rejection, the therapist summarizes and evokes Saul's emotional reality and asks him if he sees his own small, pressured self. He responds,

"No, I can't see him—his face—he is a ghost." The therapist reflects and repeats and validates that indeed Saul disappeared and lost himself to try to please those he longed to connect with, which was impossible. All routes led to pain and loss. Staying there, the therapist suggests that his small self is afraid. He comments that it is "hell" being a ghost and then is able to move into seeing this vulnerable part of himself as terrified of being labeled a traitor, and so becoming invisible. The drama moves into the now balanced adult Saul being able to tell his young self, "You must live, whatever the price. Get out. Try." This felt like an emotional epiphany, and it began in Session 11.

In the last session, Saul announces that he has started to share more with his partner and that they have decided to seek EFT couple therapy. He laughs and comments, "I get now that my partner is not my mother. I can tell her that I need space." He also notes that his dark periods of depression have vastly improved, that he is dealing with his physical pain much better and has found ways for his conservation work to really take off and become recognized. He tells the therapist, "You somehow found a way to follow and clarify the chaotic plot behind all this pain, and I can now see me and feel compassion for myself."

Recalling the early session where he outlined his self disgust and all his failings, he particularly noted that the therapist had simply said, "Of course," and then proceeded to outline how this was all perfectly logical, given that he was never seen or accepted as a child or adolescent. The therapist then laid out how it was his pattern of pain and shame that imprisoned him. He had been shocked and had refused this formulation, stating very emphatically that this was "heresy" and the therapist had laughed and agreed, saying that this way of seeing was new and was breaking all the rules he had grown up with and internalized. The therapist remembered this too and commented that Saul liked philosophy so much and that "heresy" is a word filled with religious values—with judgments about what is true and sacred. Heresy is dangerous and leads to damnation; and indeed, to be rejected and alone or told to pay an impossible price for any connection does threaten our very survival as emotional bonding human beings. The therapist then validated (Move 5) Saul's intensity and the courage he had found to aim high and try to live an intense life. He laughed and commented that he doesn't need to hide anymore, and that he felt he could be intense in therapy. One of his last comments was that "the bombs have been defused" and he was "not afraid of the anguish inside me anymore."

Saul came to therapy as a wounded war vet but in fact, as with so many such clients, the impacts of his military experiences were vastly magnified by the attachment injuries of his childhood and the expectations he had when he joined the military—that he would finally belong.

This was the path not only to a sense of belonging, but to be part of a band of strong heroes and brothers with the sacred purpose of protecting his homeland and his loved ones, and this would then soothe the ache in his heart. He left the military limping and feeling an outcast and a failure but now has found a new way to be Saul and a new path to belonging.

It was a privilege to work with him.

PLAY AND PRACTICE

For You Personally

Most trauma clients see themselves as somehow at fault for their anguish. When do you judge yourself most harshly? Try to think of a specific incident where this judgment took you over. See if you can use the steps of Affect Assembly to tune into this experience.

How did you/do you find a way out of this harsh self-judgment and back to balance and self-acceptance?

If there is no way out, what do you do to try to deal with your self-judgment? Again, try to be specific. Often, the ways we find to escape our pain lead straight back into the maze of despair.

How do the elements above relate to your experience of attachment relationships in your life?

For You Professionally

Saul was a very intellectual, intense client. How do you find yourself challenged by such clients?

Find a place in the transcript above where you might have gotten stuck and become frustrated. Consider what the therapist did and if and how it might fit for you.

We often use a Move 5 summary when we get stuck in therapy or are unsure of best next steps. What is your default option when you become confused or unsure in therapy, or wish to redirect the client to maintain momentum?

How do you deepen the client's emotional engagement when they enter into the on-target zone?

What is the main thing that you learned from reading this chapter?

KEY TAKEAWAYS

Focusing the Session and Maintaining Momentum

Avoid rabbit holes (e.g., following when the client exits; see also *A Primer for EFIT,* Johnson & Campbell, 2022).

Lead and follow.

- *Lead* the client into and through emotion.
- *Prompt* with open-ended questions such as, "What are you drawn to do?"; "What might you say?"
- *Follow* when emotion or felt experience takes hold. Trust the power and potency of attachment.

Summarize and reflect to remain on target.
Redirect as needed.
Structure the session to make the most of it.
Use the EFT Tango as a guide.
Use self of therapist (e.g., tone of voice and presence) to maintain focus and momentum.
Bolster and resource the client to build capacity.
When client exits, validate to contextualize, ensure the client feels seen and heard, then refocus as appropriate.
When interruption is needed to maintain focus, preface with rationale, then redirect. Maintain a collaborative stance.
Transparency facilitates collaboration and choice. When you feel the client's hesitation or resistance, validate and convey the intent of the intervention(s).
Keep your eye on the target. Persist and repeat. Maintain focus.

7

Harnessing Connection to Dissolve Shame in Stage 2

What is shame? To answer this question, we turn again to attachment science, the attachment view of health, and to the EFT Tango. Relationally, shame is an inhibitor—it blocks connection. For years, we have heard partners in couple relationships say some version of, "You hear everything I say as criticism." "I compliment you. I praise what you do, but you don't hear me, you don't take it in." "I can't reach you." "Where are you, where are you, where are you?" In short, for these people, the answer to the central questions surrounding a secure (ARE; Accessible, Responsive, Engaged) relationship, "Are you there for me?" "Can I count on you?" "Will you be there for me when I need you?" "Do you reach for me?" and "Do you need and rely on me?" is either a resounding or equivocal, "No." In either case, not an answer that offers a felt sense of security.

Similarly, when we have tracked couple interactions with the EFT Tango, corresponding observations emerge. At the outset of therapy, clients stuck in shame often do not look at their loved ones. They shrink and retreat, lower their eyes, turn away. As therapy proceeds in Stage 1 and bonding moments are choreographed by the therapist, especially in Moves 2 and 3 of the Tango, these partners struggle to access their inner emotional worlds and share. They struggle to take in the warmth and vulnerability of their partners (Move 4 of the Tango). Not because they do not want to, of course, but because they are blocked from doing so.

Shame blocks connection, but it also blocks access to self and inner experience. As viewed through the lens of attachment, the EFT therapist understands, translates, and distills these interactional patterns into some version of, "I can't see you if you're not to be seen. I can't know you if you're not to be known." Another translation might be something like, "I can't share that which I don't know. I am lost and alone." In other words, the withdrawal response is not withholding, but without access.

In the individual therapy space, we have similarly, for years, heard our clients say, "I don't know who I am. I feel disconnected, numb, detached, outside my body, dead." Congruent with such descriptors, clinical and interpersonal observations in such circumstances might include expressionless faces, constricted breathing, hurried speech, reactive anger, or some combination of any such process elements. Again, conceptualized through the lens of attachment, we view these process-based observations as indications of insecure attachment, that is, shutting down, reactively intensifying emotion, or some combination of both. We recognize distance from self and experience as a survival mechanism in intolerable circumstances, but also as a barrier to ongoing and healthy development of a coherent and integrated sense of self, especially when layers of shame are involved, and particularly when prototypical strategies have become automatic and reflexive.

How do we use these observations and an attachment lens to guide our understanding of shame? What are the central assumptions that help us join with and validate our clients' prototypical responses, and make sense of the interactional patterns we so commonly observe in couple therapy, or hear about in individual therapy sessions?

SHAME CAN BE ADAPTIVE IN CERTAIN CIRCUMSTANCES

When considered in context, the action tendency connected to shame (e.g., to hide, retreat, withdraw, react with anger) can be adaptive, when distance offers safety. It is adaptive to shrink and turn away in caregiving environments typified by danger, abuse, neglect, or deprivation. For example, "If I hold my breath and am very quiet, store my shoes perfectly aligned and in the right place, and do all my chores, maybe my dad won't . . . " or, "If I stay really still, retreat into the bed sheets, my dresser lodged against my bedroom door, maybe . . . " Shame is the prototypical adaptive response when key others, from whom we expect care and love, instead violate, abandon, and betray us. Shame responses are most likely to take hold and become entrenched especially when these sorts of damaging caregiver desertions occur early in development and are chronic and/or cumulative. As Sierra conveyed in an earlier chapter, in the context of deprivation, loss, and trauma, she mostly felt alone and invisible, at times as though she "didn't exist." When there is no place to belong or be cared for, it is adaptive to remain hidden.

A shame response might also be adaptive in circumstances that consistently engender a sense of helplessness, overwhelm, or inadequacy, or in situations involving what has been described as *survivor guilt* or *moral injury* (e.g., see Knobloch & Owens, 2024). A sense of feeling undeserving might ensue, even punishment or retribution. The more the sense of self becomes engulfed in shame, the greater the likelihood of self-loathing and an associated propensity to withdraw and retreat in relationships, the very relationships that might offer fertile ground for an ever-evolving coherent sense of self. Again, translated and understood through the lens of attachment, the EFT therapist hears, for example, "If I reveal myself, most certainly you will see just how damaged/defective/despicable [any of a variety of such negative descriptors might apply] I am, and you will reject me." Herein lies the existential dilemma, do I dare risk revealing myself, or is it better to be alone? The latter option invariably stalls growth and is inherently traumatizing, thus leading to a self-perpetuating cycle of distress and isolation.

SHAME COLORS THE SENSE OF SELF AS BAD

The self-definition surrounding shame is adaptive when bad things are happening and we are powerless. It is better to believe it is us, than to believe otherwise. This provides some semblance of control and predictability, and a glimmer of hope that specific actions or self-improvement of some kind might lead to better consequences.

When we are young, our need for connection is not just hardwired, it is a biological imperative, a matter of life and death. In the context of deprivation or abuse, young children have limited ways to manage. One of the solutions is to believe, "I am bad, I must be bad, if only . . . " and to block the hardwired basic need for love and acceptance.

To conclude there is something wrong with oneself is much better than the pain of longing in a famine of felt security. There is a moment of control in that. It operates as a temporary survival mechanism, an affect regulation strategy. To again refer to Sierra, it gets us through the night, when we are literally alone in the dark, however, it does not work if we get stuck there—a means of protection becomes a prison.

EARLY CUMULATIVE EXPERIENCES
OF SHAME THWART DEVELOPMENT

In the absence of any refuge outside a neglectful or traumatic caregiving environment, shame becomes automatic and reflexive and begins to define and constrict the sense of self. When the characteristic response to bad things happening becomes self-blame, or when the most adaptive response is to somehow distance from the emotion linked to the experience, the opportunity to learn and grow is obstructed. Self-resources and energy turn to vigilance for threat rather than discovery and exploration. Opportunities to learn in school are instead met with inattention, even dissociation. Navigation of peer and adult relationships through the developmental years becomes restricted by emotional responses (e.g., numbing out, lashing out) that turn people away or shut others out. Labels from others become self-defining. Rejection leads to further self-deprecation and self-blame. Further withdrawal leads to increased fear and mistrust. Self-destructive strategies to cope become reliable and relied upon (e.g., addictions, self-harm behaviors such as cutting, disordered eating), leading individuals further away from themselves and others. Self-perpetuating patterns of distress and distancing further add to the layers of armour that block access to self, and connection with others.

In circumstances involving chronic or cumulative trauma exposure, self-loathing and self-blame are likely to become more firmly entrenched, and the prototypical shame response becomes increasingly automatic and reflexive. Over time, access to self and experience is consistently blocked, along with connection to others. Growth is thwarted. Shame eclipses the sense of self. The world becomes dark and dangerous, and the way out unclear. Joseph, stuck in the past and in a vicious cycle of rotating relationships, felt trapped. "Each time I think I found the love and approval I never had, I mess it up, then crumble into long periods of substance abuse and depression, crawl back out of that hole, then do it again. What's the point? I'm a loser, destined to fail and to be alone."

FINDING THE WAY OUT OF SHAME
AND INTO GROWTH AND CONNECTION

Repair is possible. We are all vulnerable to a shame response. We share the propensity to retreat to avoid rejection or disapproval following what we (or critical others) perceive as a mistake or transgression, but this is especially so if our earlier experiences have led us to perceive ourselves as somehow bad or unworthy. Shame (and its close relative, guilt) is the common response to some type of mistake or transgression and is adaptive when it then leads to interpersonal repair, compassion, and/or some type of forgiveness, of self or other(s).

We know from our AIRM (Attachment Injury Resolution Model) protocol that shame can be a barrier to fully engaging with the expression of a partners' pain, and to fully engaging with and expressing a sincere apology (e.g., see Halchuk, Makinen, & Johnson, 2010; Johnson, Makinen, & Millikin, 2001; Makinen & Johnson, 2006; Naaman et al., 2005). We also recognize that as shame is dissolved in this Stage 2 process of couple therapy, access to self-experience is gained, allowing for an authentic expression of regret, as well as an increased capacity to be with and accept the pain and vulnerability of a key other. The relationship is transformed, as are both partners within it.

Personal strengths, such as intellect as in the case of Sierra, might light and provide a path forward out of shame and into growth and resilience. Key others may also lend a helping hand, though with limited benefit if the individual is unable to take it in, or to accept the love, care, and respect of another. In some cases, often depending on the degree to which prior relational experiences have been marked by events such as betrayal or abandonment and the sense of self has become entrenched in shame, strengths and social resources may challenge the prevailing self-view, facilitate self-compassion, and similarly begin to shift view of other. In other cases, however, the individual might be unable to find compassion for self or accept the loving gaze of a key other without the support of a trusted clinician and effective therapeutic method.

EFT offers a roadmap and a method. With the three-stage process and key interventions reviewed in earlier chapters, we now focus on how we address shame, specifically in Stage 2 of EFCT. Building on and with consideration given to what was outlined above, the following is a collection of considerations and assumptions central to our understanding and treatment of shame, along with a therapy transcript involving a couple relationship impacted by personal and intimate relationship trauma. As in other chapters, the transcript will include therapist commentary.

KEY ASSUMPTIONS FOR TREATING SHAME IN EFT

Shame Is Relational: Change Happens in Relationship

Close relatives of shame such as embarrassment, humiliation, and guilt are similarly relational. When such descriptors emerge in the therapy process, we recognize their proximity and relevance in understanding the key role of shame on a developing sense of self, and the corresponding goal of EFT for couples and for individuals—to directly and explicitly restructure self and system (Stage 2). Just as shame develops and evolves in relationship, so too does change occur. Change is inherently interpersonal in nature, sculpted by the emotional messages that occur in dialogue with another.

Proximity to Self Offers a Starting Point and Can Be a Gauge of Progress

For clients who have felt invisible in their early years, this same experience often occurs around attempts to get close to their younger, more vulnerable selves. Blank canvases emerge, possibly shadows, profiles, faceless figures, or the backs of a younger more vulnerable self. Saul, for example, caught in the bind of shame and rejection, in early sessions, had little to no access to his younger, more vulnerable self: "I can't see him—his face—he is a ghost." Once again, such responses are understood as manifestations of adaptation in earlier circumstances and are validated in context. Interventions are titrated with respect to ongoing assessment of capacity and flexibility, and with attention to personal, self, and social resources both within and outside the therapy process. Progress is observed such that as contact with bodily felt or emotional experience increases, so too does access to self.

Emotion Links Self and Experience

Disconnecting from one's inner emotional or felt experience, through numbing or reactive intensification, leads to disconnection from self. In the case of trauma, and especially longstanding trauma exposure, when the only choice is to emotionally remove oneself from intolerable experience, distance from self and experience broadens, and access shrinks. Emotion, as manifested and expressed in various forms across individuals, families, communities, and cultures, is the way home. Most typically, ready access is unavailable, and it is the bodily felt experience that provides the gateway to previously disavowed emotionally charged experiences likely to have been pivotal in shaping self-perceptions and dances with others.

Stillness Facilitates Immediacy

Contacting bodily felt experience or emotional experience, distilling and ordering it, and then sharing it coherently and directly with a reliable attachment figure is the key mechanism of change in EFT. As alluded to in earlier chapters, attachment security and the capacity to engage with self and emotion can be viewed on a continuum. For some, capacity and access to self might be highly limited in the early sessions of Stage 1. For others, they might have more capacity and flexibility with previously relied upon strategies for managing distress. Regardless of strategy (numbing out, reactive intensification, or a mixed combination), distance from self and experience is the natural consequence. Initial goals then, following the creation of a safe haven alliance, the experiential process-based assessment, and the identification and magnification of resources, are to increase proximity. Whether our clients are reactively intensifying emotion, shutting it down, or a mixed combination, stillness is the way home, to self and experience. When we ask our clients to tune into themselves and their experience, be still with their bodies and their inner worlds, something inevitably emerges. Felt shifts occur when these emotional realities are shared with a safe other(s). For example, as demonstrated in the chapter featuring Sierra, "I don't feel anything," shifted to, "fear or vacancy," to "fear" and when seen and heard by another, Sierra felt "relief"—a corrective emotional experience.

Shame Is Contextualized in Stage 1 through Tracking, Reflection, and Validation

The target of change in EFT is not shame per se, but instead, access to (Stage 1) and, ultimately, restructuring of view of self (Stage 2). In the first stage of therapy, we are essentially challenging prototypical responses, the action tendency for shame. Said differently, we are helping clients move from automaticity and rigidity to flexibility in response, broadening the space between trigger and response (more about this below). In Stage 2, we are confronting the shame-infused definition of self. In Stage 1, shame may or may not be explicitly acknowledged by the therapist but is recognized as key in the therapy process and, as appropriate, validated and contextualized in the client's narrative. Again, validation offers a means of contextualizing prototypical responses and such interventions are titrated based on capacity. For example, for the individual therapy client completely unable to see or contact felt experience and/or view of self, the therapist might say, "It makes sense. Of course it is hard to get close to you and your inner emotional world, your felt experience. It was not safe to do so in earlier times. Your best recourse was to shut down, and shut others out, but the problem with this, of course, over time, is that it has left you alone. Now, when you have a partner you perceive as a safe other, it is hard to get close, to trust, and it is hard to believe or accept the love your partner tries to provide. Is that right? Am I getting this right?" For others, who might name their shame, or whose sense of self is not engulfed in multiple layers of shame based on an accumulation of shame-evoking experiences, the therapist might reflect, "I hear you. Every time you get close to sharing some aspect of your past, shame emerges, and your tendency is to retreat. That was the adaptive move in earlier times. But now this strategy of shutting down and hiding is leaving you feeling alone and lonely, and what I hear you say is you don't know how to escape this trap. This is good. The more you can begin to see yourself and your experience in earlier times, the easier it will be to move forward from those experiences. You can do this; you're doing it now." As highlighted here and elsewhere in our writings, the focus of validation is on the shame *response* (hiding, retreating, withdrawing, lashing out), not the *outcome* (feelings of worthlessness and failure). We reflect that which we want our clients to notice. Attention is not drawn to the shame-infused definition of self, but is mentally noted by the therapist, and is a key target of change.

Compassion Is the Antidote

In initial sessions, validating statements such as those above are aimed at helping clients feel seen and heard so that they can begin to hear and see themselves in new ways, specifically surrounding shame, with some compassion. Compassion is the antidote to shame and self-denigration, to self-loathing and self-blame, and to a reflexive tendency to shut down and shut out.

Prototypical Responses Shift from Rigidity to Flexibility

As access and capacity to embody self and experience expands, so too does flexibility. The space between trigger and response widens. Increased access and flexibility, key areas of change in Stage 1, provide the foundation for deeper level change in Stage 2. Specifically, it allows for the dissolution of shame and the restructuring of self, and complimentary restructuring of system, that is, how we relate to others. As described elsewhere, being leads to belonging. When clients take the risk of tuning in and sharing themselves with key others, acceptance of self and other and a sense of belonging become possible.

As Access to Self and Experience Expands, Shame Dissolves

With increased capacity and flexibility, the therapist can guide the client into deeper levels of experience for longer periods, more directly access and reshape the shame-infused self, and choreograph engaged encounters at deeper levels of experience. Numerous EFT couple therapy process and outcome studies have highlighted the importance of level of experiencing in creating the type of change we described earlier as second order change, and that characterizes change in Stage 2 (Myung, Furrow, & Lee, 2022; Spengler et al., 2024). In short, these studies have used the level of experiencing scale (Klein et al., 1969) as a measure to demonstrate that deep and sustainable gains (that restructure attachment) occur when clients are able to access experience at Levels 4 and above (Kailanko, S. et al., 2022). That is, when clients can move into and be absorbed by experience, rather than talking about it, as is the case in lower levels, such as Levels 1 and 2 on the Experiencing Scale. It is at this level of experiencing that the self is most readily accessed, that negative views of self and other can be confronted and reshaped in deep and sustainable ways, and that change leads to *identity epiphanies* and capacity for deep connection, bonding. The natural consequence of increased access to and opportunity for restructuring—from negative to positive, constricted to expanded, insecure to secure—is the dissolution of shame.

RESTRUCTURING SELF IN RELATIONSHIP IN STAGE 2

Research and clinical wisdom guide the order of intervention surrounding the two key change events in Stage 2 couple therapy, withdrawer engagement first, followed by pursuer softening. Indeed, most reassuring for any partner seeking contact and closeness is the felt presence of a key other, that is, contact with an authentic self, expanded and exposed, no longer shrouded by shame. The complementary consequence for the revealing partner is opportunity, in real time, to not only be seen and heard, but embraced and accepted, loved and lovable—being and belonging, the story of development—growth through connection. As couples gain access to themselves and each other in new, deeper ways, not only does their bond deepen, so too does their capacity to grow and evolve in their most important relationship—with each other!

A parallel process occurs in the individual therapy context. As capacity increases over the course of Stage 1, the client can move into deeper levels of experience for longer periods. Trust and access build in Stage 1 individual therapy, just as it does in the first stage of EFT couple therapy. As trust and safety to explore, discover, and regain disavowed aspects of self and experience increases, indications of de-escalation (the Stage 1 change event in couple therapy), such as less conflict, become evident, along with indications of personal growth of partners within the relationship, specifically, increased trust and access/capacity. Similarly, in the individual therapy realm, various indicators of increased proximity to self and experience become apparent. A fundamental difference in individual and couple therapy, of course, is the physical absence of a key attachment figure in the therapy space. As described elsewhere, however, there are a cast of characters that live in the minds and hearts of our clients, and that have been engaged in the therapy process, as seen with Sierra and her grandmother, and an older, wiser, more resourced self. Often, as demonstrated in earlier chapters, the therapist harnesses the power of the relationship with self to move clients toward a greater felt sense of security with themselves and others, with the understanding that sustainable gains within session will inevitably generalize to relationships outside of therapy. In other terms, once the organic growth process is kick-started, clients will continue to grow and evolve in their most important relationships (Johnson & Campbell, 2022).

Late in the Stage 1 individual therapy process (Session 12 in this case), Sandy revisited a scene involving sexual exploitation and violation, representative of many that had been instrumental in shaping attachment. At this point, not only was she able to get close to her younger, more vulnerable 9-year-old self, she was able to be in her body—to feel what was intolerable and unsafe to feel at the time of the traumatic incident. In contrast, early encounters with her older, wiser, more resourced self were met with disdain and disappointment, rejection and mistrust. She was angry and resentful, resolved to remain shut off and shut down.

By Session 12, increased trust and emotional capacity and flexibility had been gained, along with proximity. The details of the scene made vivid (not the traumatic incident), emotion was intense and level of experiencing deep. As the therapist dimmed the threat (i.e., the perpetrator) to avoid any possibility of retraumatization and to maintain focus and momentum, the more vulnerable aspect of self (the child in the scene) was supported to continue to engage deeply with the vulnerability she had adaptively disembodied in earlier times. In contrast, the presence of relational resources was illuminated, her older, wiser, more resourced adult self in the foreground, and the therapist in the background.

Propelled and guided by the power and potency of attachment, her older, wiser, more resourced self organically entered the scene, assertively removed her younger vulnerable self, and took her to safety.

As this powerful encounter unfolded and was processed, various indications of shame emerged, such as the embarrassment of feeling like she asked for it because she kept going back. In each instance, the older, wiser adult self was invited to respond (assumed to be much more powerful than the therapist responding) and was able to directly and firmly confront the underpinnings of various ways of being and relating. At one point, she vehemently declared, "It's not your fault." With access to self and experience up and running, the therapist directed her to repeat it. She did so, and added, "It's not your fault. This is something being done to you." Move 4 inquiries revealed capacity to take it in, restructure and reshape self, and by extension, dissolve shame.

As this and other Stage 2 changes occurred, Sandy expressed and exhibited increased confidence and competence. She also began to share her internal needs, fears, vulnerabilities, and longings with those who matter most, her "perfect partner," her sister and her mother, and as importantly, she began to take in—and believe in—the love and admiration they had been providing for years prior. The organic growth process kick-started, a more positive sense of self continued to evolve in her most important relationships.

GRIEF NATURALLY EMERGES AS CLIENTS GAIN NEW ACCESS TO SECURE ATTACHMENT

In the face of overwhelming distress, especially early in development, the only recourse is to somehow shut down, disavow aspects of self and experience, and adapt in the face of threat and trauma. As individuals find safety and security in the arms of trusted and trustworthy others, and come home to themselves, the magnitude of the loss incurred inevitably surfaces. Most certainly, not all loss involves trauma, but all trauma, especially developmental trauma, involves loss. The inevitable grief process is honored as integral to ongoing progress, making space for something or someone new, including new aspects of self and experience, anticipated to continue to emerge in an ever-evolving sense of self in relationship, and an ever-evolving relationship.

RESTRUCTURING SELF AND SYSTEM IN STAGE 2 COUPLE THERAPY: A CASE EXAMPLE

Informed by the above principles, we now introduce you to a couple and offer a window into the Stage 2 couple therapy process. You will notice that the Tango is applied with couples, just as it is with individuals, the main difference being the choreographed encounter between partners, rather than an imaginal other. As couples begin to approach Stage 2, momentum has been gained. Increased capacity, presence, and trust have made them better Tango dancers! They are more tuned in and attuned. As with the individual therapy process, access to self and experience has broadened, along with the breadth and depth of their emotional and behavioral repertoires. Prototypical strategies for being and relating are more flexible and fluid. Deeper contact with self and other has led to increased self-compassion and compassion and understanding for others.

Such was the case for Randy and Karen, devoted to personal

growth and their marriage, they had been engaged in therapy intermittently over the past years, of various forms, including both individual and couple therapy. They had made significant progress. Nonetheless, Karen continued to long for a closer relationship. The couple was referred for a live consult by their primary therapist and was at that time presumed to be at the edge of Stage 2 but thus far unable to cross that threshold.

Some brief background information for both partners was provided by their primary therapist. Of particular relevance regarding Randy's background was that his father was a military veteran, had served overseas, and was, to cite Randy, likely suffering from unrecognized and untreated PTSD. Whatever the case, Randy's reality in early childhood was one of unpredictability, abuse, and trauma. Seen through the eyes of an innocent little boy, his father was a tyrant. He had recalled numerous poignant memories of his mother being terrorized, chased around their bedroom as Randy hid in his own, dinner table scenes ending in broken glass, and long cold silences as Randy walked from the pantry to his father's favorite chair with his regular dose of scotch. According to his therapist, one such experience seemed to emerge often in therapy, an incident involving his father's rage, leaving Randy and his mother locked out of the family home and shivering in the snow.

The couple was in their early 20s when they started dating. Randy had shared that meeting Karen was a blessing, and most certainly changed the trajectory of his life. By then, Randy had struggled with various forms of addiction, as well as long and severe bouts of depression. Suicidal ideation and an attempt in adolescence also marked his history. Her history was much different. A nice home, loving parents, and well on her way in a health-related career. Her developmental history was characterized as secure, their therapist explained. Their relationship had been tumultuous at various times over the years, sometimes on the brink of breakup, and most certainly scarred by multiple attachment injuries, that is, experiences of betrayal or abandonment.

According to their therapist, the grip that various forms of addiction once had on Randy and their relationship had been successfully addressed. Their relationship was much less tumultuous than it had been in prior years. However, echoes of Randy's developmental trauma continued to pulse through his body, his shame remained a barrier to self and connection, and personal and relational wounds prevailed for both partners. The transcript (edited for brevity) of the session provided below represents the shift from Stage 1 into Stage 2 and demonstrates a key Stage 2 change event in EFT for couples—withdrawer engagement—a precursor and concomitant factor in the dissolution of shame when part-ners are facing trauma together.

THERAPIST: It's my understanding, Randy, that you've done a huge amount of work over the years, and you have been together for a long time?

KAREN: We have.

RANDY: Yes, we're celebrating our 35th anniversary.

THERAPIST: So nice. Do you guys notice the way you look at each other? [Therapist draws attention to process elements, specifically rela-tional capacity.]

KAREN: No.

THERAPIST: It's very beautiful.

KAREN: Yeah?

RANDY: Well, we've been through a lot, but we've continued to perse-vere, and Karen's been very supportive. Literally, I wouldn't be here today if it wasn't for her and the help that I've had along the way.

THERAPIST: That's nice, that's touching. So, to go back, did you talk about what you hope to gain from coming? Do you have a goal or something that you've talked about? [The therapist is focusing on creating safety but also attending to view of self as linked with the current and recurring symptom picture, specifically, anxiety and depression.]

RANDY: Well, I'll maybe start off and then, Karen, you can add whatever you want. I've been really struggling with confidence and feeling worthy, and when I go out into the real world and start interacting, my insecurities come through and they take me to some pretty dark places at times. I've come a long way. I'm somewhat better, but. . . . Would you like to add to that, Karen? I'm not too good at describ-ing things like that. From your point of view, what do you think?

KAREN: I think that's true, and yes, he's been struggling more than ever in the last little while with heightened anxiety. Our therapist is say-ing that it's because he's now starting to get in touch with his feel-ings, so he's feeling all these things, but it's becoming quite difficult for him to navigate lately. I was trying to tell him about what I was learning from your website last night. It would be great if we could learn something about attachment—it would help to sort of allevi-ate that anxiety. I had seen that video, with the woman who had done the MRI and the brain activity. [Here Karen is referencing the

MRI study, demonstrating that secure attachment can soothe the nervous system of an anxious partner; Coan et al., 2006; Johnson et al., 2013].

THERAPIST: Yes, good for you! Excellent! That's so nice! Do you hear what she's saying, Randy?

RANDY: Yes.

THERAPIST: "I would like to help you to heal those wounds through our attachment." That's what you said. (*Looking at Karen.*) That's great.

RANDY: Basically, I'm living in a constant state of anxiety, and I'm dealing with it now without having to depend on my typical escape.

THERAPIST: Yeah, what is your typical escape? [Therapist is inquiring about prototypical attachment strategy.]

RANDY: Well, I've done everything . . .

THERAPIST: Oh, okay. So, what does that mean?

RANDY: I've done the alcohol thing. I've done the porn thing. I've done the prostitute thing. I've done the eating thing.

THERAPIST: And now, how do you escape? Or do you?

RANDY: Uhm, I'm learning to. I still feel a lot of it and there's times when my anxiety is bad; I can't escape it, you know? And sometimes I'm learning to talk to Karen and to depend on her but it's so foreign to me to do that. It certainly hasn't been natural; I tune out naturally and go into my own little world.

THERAPIST: And then what do you do, Karen, when he goes into his own little world. What happens for you? [Therapist is inquiring about relational impact of this attachment strategy/delineating the cycle.]

KAREN: I usually get frustrated. I try to push my way through, and then sometimes I give up and then give him the silent treatment. I do all kinds of things just to try to connect. Sometimes we talk into all hours of the night, it might get escalated at first, and sometimes, I can reach through, into a crack and see the real him. I can kind of pull him along a little bit. [Karen describes our earlier description, "shame eclipses the self" and notes that she can sometimes find her partner through a crack.]

THERAPIST: Karen, what does that mean when you say, "I can see the real him?" [Therapist hears this as, "I can see his authentic self." The key goal in EFT is to bring clients home to themselves, to their internal worlds, to afford them flexibility to tune into their inner emotional worlds, their needs, fears, longings, vulnerabilities and share with key trusted others—to grow and thrive in their most important relationships. Karen's experience provides an indicator of where the couple is in the process.]

KAREN: What it means is that he shuts down, he disengages.

THERAPIST: But he peeks through the cracks, is that when you see the real him?

KAREN: Sometimes I can see. You know, the way he looks or the way he reacts, or just what he says. I can see that we've made a little tiny spark of a connection, and then we sort of try to walk through that. But yeah, it can be frustrating. I think a lot of times, I just trigger him.

THERAPIST: Is she triggering you now?

RANDY: It's always uncomfortable to hear about stuff like that, yeah.

THERAPIST: When she said, "I trigger him," I maybe didn't understand it. Maybe that's a good place to explore a bit more? When Karen reaches to you, Randy, and you're in a place where you don't want to be reached or maybe don't even feel like you're in reach of yourself, is that accurate? What is happening for you, internally, when Karen is reaching to you? [The therapist is bringing forth the negative cycle they get stuck in as a means of anchoring the process, building an alliance, and beginning to focus the session. Notice also that the therapist highlights the understanding that withdrawing partners are not necessarily withholding but rather unable to share that which they do not have access to. That is, their internal emotional worlds, a common sequela of developmental/complex trauma.]

RANDY: Well, sometimes it feels so painful, and when I reach the point that I feel there's no hope, it's hard for her to penetrate me—I just want to retreat into my own little hellhole. At that point I don't feel that anything can make a difference.

THERAPIST: Is that what you did as a kid, Randy? Is that childhood-based? [Developmental considerations are again key, longstanding adaptive strategies are often more rigid and automatic/reflexive.]

RANDY: Yes, it is, and I've come to understand through therapy that in order to cope, or survive, what I did was just go into my own little world. It was so natural for me. It's just what I did, and now I can identify it.

THERAPIST: Right, you notice it, and understand it.

RANDY: Yes, those things were my norm. I didn't know anything different. I just knew something was wrong with me. [Therapist hears view of self at the forefront, "something wrong with me," the natural consequence of a childhood characterized by trauma, abandonment and neglect, combined with isolation.]

THERAPIST: So now, Randy, today, what do you feel, in your eyes, at various times in our interaction together? [As the therapist tracks process elements, notably glassy/teary eyes at times, attention is directed to signs of connection with self and experience in the here and now.]

RANDY: I get sad. There's nothing happy about it, and there's a lot of time in one's life that's wasted. I just get sad when I get into these conversations. [The therapist hears indications of loss and hopelessness.]

THERAPIST: Yes, loss, is that it? When you say, "time wasted," you're referencing a feeling of loss? [Reflecting that which we want the client to notice, or draw attention to, loss versus hopelessness, as the goal is to engender hope as the session progresses.]

RANDY: Yes, loss, there has been a lot of loss. I don't know what to say now. (*Randy turns to his wife.*)

THERAPIST: It's okay, this is perfect. What I'm aware of, Randy, is that you've done lots of amazing, beautiful work with your therapist, and I'm this new person coming in and I feel like I'm catching up. So, I'm just trying to hear from you about your experience. I think you are both so beautifully articulate. What I'm mostly struck by is just how you look at one another, it's so nice. [Once again, the therapist draws attention to process elements, in this case, specifically the connection between the couple, and possible signs of de-escalation, the first key change event in EFT couple therapy.]

RANDY: Sometimes it hasn't been. . . . I'm very lucky to have Karen, and I love her, but sometimes I get angry at her, too.

THERAPIST: And sometimes you still hide, is what I hear?

RANDY: Yes.

THERAPIST: And you retreat into this place, you call it your "hellhole." Is it a hellhole? What happens in this place and space? [Therapist begins to explore what happens when Randy retreats, not to focus on and/or highlight dark moods or experiences, but to get closer to his inner, deeper experience.]

RANDY: It's my inner hell.

THERAPIST: Oh, I get it. Are you actually present in there, or are you sort of numb from yourself as well? [Therapist explores from a stance of curiosity, not assumption, with the intent to also encourage clients to move into self-exploration and discovery.]

RANDY: I get numb from myself as well. My therapist has been helping me to actually identify where that is, and I know it's in my inner core, so I just go back in there. Then when I go back in there, I just shut everything off, and when I get really deep in there . . . that's the place I dread, when I say, "There's nothing worth living for."

THERAPIST: And are you at risk for suicide at those times, or not so much? Or have you been?

RANDY: I have been in the past.

THERAPIST: Currently, or not so much now? [The therapist considers the capacity of the relationship, as well as each partner within it, to gauge progress to date, and to guide the pacing of interventions and the possible goals for this consult.]

RANDY: I'm going through a difficult time, with fitting in at work, and I'm feeling, a lot, that I don't measure up. At times, I just get these feelings that everybody's out to get me, that I'm not good enough, and I keep trying and trying. Karen, what do you think? What do I do? [Therapist notices indicators of view of self and other: vigilance for threat and disapproval, and an ongoing propensity to find confirming evidence; no sense of belonging; and a tendency to look outward, that is, to defer to others rather than trust and rely on self and inner experience.]

KAREN: I think you're avoiding the question.

RANDY: Yeah . . .

KAREN: It's been a rough go, the last week or two.

THERAPIST: Oh, okay. Are you worried about him? [Therapist also turns to partner to gauge safety.]

KAREN: I am worried about him, yeah.

THERAPIST: Randy, are you worried about you in that regard? Do you feel hopeless right now? [Therapist is tuning in and finding focus, while also assessing for safety, personally and relationally, and attending to creating a "safe haven" therapeutic alliance.]

RANDY: I'm not. I don't get worried.

THERAPIST: No, you go numb you said, you shut down.

RANDY: There's a lot happening now, but I just don't feel that I'm good enough, and I feel that I want to be recognized, sometimes I so desperately want to be recognized. But no matter what I try to do . . . my organization's gone through a major review, and I've worked hard, and I've tried to do things, but I never seem to get selected for advancement. I'm doing okay, but it's not where I'd like to be. I truly believe that I'm not good enough. I don't like to face it, but . . . [View of self is at the forefront.]

THERAPIST: That's the place where your brain goes, yeah? (*Randy responds affirmatively.*)

KAREN: And he's at this low state, where I was talking to him about opioid-induced hyperalgesia, where, when you're taking opioids, not only do you develop tolerance, but your pain threshold actually lessens, and I said, "That's almost what's happened to you, it's not opioid-induced, but you're hypersensitive." Somebody can laugh and he'll think it's directed at him, or they'll laugh at him, but he really thinks it's humiliating. That's a really hard place to be. [Karen is highlighting some of the interpersonal impacts of these core attachment elements, view of self and other, and attachment strategy and capacity. All interactions are filtered through his template for self and other. Karen's choice of the word "humiliating" is noteworthy as a close relative of shame.]

THERAPIST: Yes, absolutely, and does it happen in your relationship? [Therapist recognizes that the past is alive in the present and has far reaching impacts but brings the discussion back to the relationship to keep focusing the session, and to continue to rely on the best-known resource we have, each other.]

KAREN: You have to answer that, Randy.

RANDY: Yeah. In our relationship, I guess when I'm feeling good, I feel like we're on par and it's just very natural, but then, like right now, I feel that I'm not good enough and so I often feel that Karen's better than me, smarter than me. [Therapist again hears indicators of view of self and tendency to feel "less than" in the relationship, likely contributing to and representing Randy's feeling of inadequacy in relationships, and Karen's experience of not having an equal partner in the relationship, someone she can fully trust and rely on.]

THERAPIST: And Randy, when you say those words, where do you feel that in your body? [Therapist begins to help Randy connect self with experience using the body as a gateway.]

RANDY: Uhm, well, you know, it's like, solidly in me because these things are so entrenched and yeah. I'm sorry I'm fumbling. Sometimes it's hard to answer questions. I have to think about them, you know, to really give you a good response. I just know how I'm feeling but I don't know how to articulate it. [Therapist hears Randy looking for the "correct" answer and is reminded of the message partners often convey in such circumstances, "I don't want you to agree with me/defer to me/tell me what you think I want to hear, I want you to be with me."]

THERAPIST: Randy, you know what? I think you're doing an amazing job. It's perfect, it's great. From my point of view, this is super help-ful. A lot of what EFT is about and what we do is to help people explore and discover and make sense of experiences that wouldn't have been safe to explore in other contexts, especially for people who have had difficult childhoods. There would be no room for that, so the best strategy for a difficult childhood environment is to shut down or to act out or do a combination of the two, but cer-tainly not to be fully present in the room because that's dangerous. That's too dangerous so somehow you have to shield yourself, some-how, some way. I don't know you very well, I'm only here for a few minutes, but the strong feeling I have is that it's just what your beau-tiful wife said. That it's an opportunity in a connected relationship and it's also all about timing, right? It didn't take one or two years to get to a place where that becomes an automatic strategy, and it doesn't take one or two years to undo it either. It takes a long time, and lots and lots of courage. It's supposed to be baby steps actually. It's not supposed to be these big leaps into the deep end because that's not how we grow, that's not how we develop, and that's not how we are supposed to be nurtured as little children. So, I'm here, just to try to help make sense, as much as we can in a short period together, of your experience and your experience with your wife. I promise you there are no right answers. I don't have any answers, I'm just wanting to walk along with you, to explore and try to make sense of it all. Maybe help you to take another step in the amaz-ing journey that you've already been on, that I've heard a little bit about. [Therapist validates and provides rationale and a road map for therapy and maintains a stance of collaboration.]

RANDY: Yeah, you're so encouraging. It sounds positive and I was saying to Karen that, in my interactions, it's very lonely, like at work, it's always, you know, you don't talk to anybody and you can't. You know what I mean? And so, like, yesterday was a very difficult day for me, just the dynamics around meetings and things, and then it just builds and builds. It is a very lonely journey. People look at you, but they don't see. And one of the things that I struggle with is that sometimes I'm working, and I feel anxious, and sometimes when I get anxious, I don't think clearly, I don't process things clearly.

THERAPIST: Yeah, of course. All your resources are elsewhere. That makes sense and that's what happens with little kids in those kinds of home environments, too. They can't sit and listen in a classroom. [Therapist validates and contextualizes prototypical strategy for coping that evolved in context of intolerable circumstances.]

KAREN: Right.

THERAPIST: All their resources are somewhere else.

KAREN: Exactly.

RANDY: Yeah. I said to Karen yesterday that I can do well, you know, if somebody can give me some encouragement. I have to try and stay calm, but I do want to do well, I want to succeed, I want to grow. But the sad part about it is that I probably cannot obtain that because I feel deficient. Maybe, when I'm . . . when things are going swell, then, yeah, I can do well. [The descriptor "deficient" is noted, another powerful indicator of model of self.]

THERAPIST: You know what, Randy? It makes me think about lots of the people I work with, and I have some thoughts about maybe what we could do here together today. Karen touched on it, she said that if we could help you . . . well, she didn't say it quite this way, but basically, she said that she could be a resource to you in this journey that you're on; that it doesn't have to be a lonely journey. That's what she said earlier. The other thing that kids don't have when they come from more difficult homes is that they don't have an attachment figure that takes them to school or that they carry with them, so under times of stress or anxiety, they can kind of call upon an image of that person to feel soothed. When we don't have it in childhood, there's not much we can do about it, but in couple relationships, we can do something. It's exactly what Karen said, you don't have to be alone. And here with me today, the more that you can share, together we can discover and try to make sense of your inner experience. Maybe that's the piece of work I'm thinking that we could do. [Therapist is focusing the session, soliciting readiness and willingness to proceed in this direction, and conveying the message that we could talk about it, but it will be much more powerful to create a new experience and then talk about that experience, essentially an introduction to the Tango, a bottom-up experiential process that can then be cognitively processed, integrated, and consolidated.]

RANDY: Yes.

THERAPIST: We can just do whatever we can do today, and Karen can be a part of that. Maybe it's not going to solve the things at work, but it's going to leave you feeling less lonely in those moments.

RANDY: Yes.

THERAPIST: And in an ideal world, kids have that and then they're brave. They're braver, of course we're all braver, when we have a crowd of people behind us, right? It's way harder to be brave when we feel like a lone person on a big journey that we don't understand.

RANDY: Right, yeah. Exactly.

KAREN: That would be great. That's a great goal, right? [The process is intended to be collaborative with the goal of not only providing agency, the agency many of our clients did not have in earlier times, but also their own road map to secure attachment outside the therapy process.]

RANDY: That's a good goal.

THERAPIST: So Randy, can we just back up? It's kind of the road map, what my inquisitive, maybe intrusive at times, questions are all about. It's about helping you, and helping me and Karen, eventually, to understand more about this place that you had to live in by yourself for lots of good reasons as a little kid. More and more that space is becoming a little tiny bit porous. That's what I heard Karen say, that there's tiny little cracks at times where she can feel you and see you. And when she does feel you and see you, do you feel seen and felt and heard in those moments? [Therapist maintains focus and keeps it relational.]

RANDY: More and more, yeah, yeah. It depends on what kind of stage I'm at, you know, but yeah, I am starting to do that.

THERAPIST: So that's a good thing, right? So, what Karen was saying was that she couldn't be there for you as a little kid, when all of this came into play.

RANDY: No.

THERAPIST: She couldn't protect you then, but now, the more that the wall becomes porous and the cracks become bigger, the more that you discover and share, the more that she feels less alone in the relationship and the more you're not on this lonely journey. You are together. [Therapist highlights and focuses specifically on model of self and access, and the relational impact.]

RANDY: Yeah, yeah. It's taken a while to do that.

THERAPIST: For good reason.

RANDY: Yeah, and you know what? One of the things I could say to you is that the more you share, then how can somebody, how can she believe in me? You know? You want to look up to somebody. So okay, you sit there, and you share this, "I did that, I did this and this." How can you sit there and admire somebody? I would like her to look up to me and respect me. [The central existential dilemma for the shame shrouded self, "If I reveal myself, most certainly you will reject me, and I will forever be alone," but of course, without the risk of finding and sharing self with a potentially trustworthy other, the individual is alone, which is in itself inherently traumatizing.]

KAREN: Is that a question for me?

RANDY: Well, I said that was one of the roadblocks.

KAREN: Yeah, that is a roadblock for you, for sure.

THERAPIST: For him, yeah. Randy, we could talk a lot about that, but it won't have nearly the power that I think feeling something different would have, if we can get to that place. But of course, it's a totally legitimate and valid concern, it's a valid desire. And part of feeling respected is risking revealing yourself, right? [The therapist names the dilemma.]

RANDY: Uh huh, yes.

THERAPIST: So that's part of the roadblock for Karen, that it's hard for her to see you when you're not to be seen, when you're behind that wall. But when she gets little glimpses of you, what I hear you both say is that that's a really nice place for each of you. A place where she can feel important and special and all of those things, and you can feel what you deserve: the recognition you've been lacking a huge amount of for a really long time. [Recognizing the resource of the relationship and increased readiness to engage, the therapist highlights the block, as well as the possibility.]

RANDY: Yeah.

THERAPIST: Maybe help me to understand the wall more or the "hole," or the whatever the word is that you used to describe that place that you go into, in your chest. [Therapist focuses on the block with the aim of dissolving it and/or helping Randy come out from behind it.]

RANDY: Yes, yeah, yeah.

THERAPIST: Do you feel it now?

RANDY: Yeah, yeah, I do. You know if I open it up . . . it's something that I've always tried to avoid because I know when I get in there, it's pretty painful. My first memories are when I was very young, I'm talking even three or four, and being frightened and scared. But it's something that . . . I don't like to go there too much. [Therapist is attentive to process elements and notices that Randy appears to go elsewhere/dissociate.]

THERAPIST: Yeah, you don't like to go into the fear.

RANDY: No. But you know . . . no . . . , mmm . . . I'm hedging.

THERAPIST: When you just shared that with me about being three or four, is it okay to keep going? [Therapist tracks process elements, notes shift in eye contact, as well as a slight quiver in voice.]

RANDY: Yeah, yeah.

THERAPIST: Did you just kind of go to that place as a kid?

RANDY: Yeah. I actually get images.

THERAPIST: Yeah, I thought I saw it in your eyes. So, what do you see, Randy? What do you see? As much as you can, if you can allow yourself to go back there, with your beautiful wife here holding you and I'll stay with you as well, what do you see and feel, Randy? [Recognizing the relational and personal capacity of the client, the therapist begins to use the image to evoke experience, the experience that was intolerable / unacceptable / not safe to feel at the time of the event; Move 2 of the Tango.]

RANDY: Well, I feel afraid. You know, I always, I get this vision, I just remember bad feelings but I don't know why. I remember when we were locked out of our home, our house, my mom and I, and it was wintertime, and she kept me warm by holding me. She was crying and knocking on the door to try to get into the house, but I don't know why. [Move 1 of the Tango, a scene representative of many, and of Randy's general felt experience: alone and lonely, no comfort in a time of need.]

KAREN: You told me that your dad locked you out.

RANDY: Yeah, my father locked us out of the house.

THERAPIST: And how old were you, Randy, in that scene?

RANDY: Three or, I don't know, definitely four tops. [Age matters; attachment theory is a developmental theory and theory of personality. The therapist is curious about how long this prototypical strategy, this wall, has been in place, and when, developmentally, these key pivotal experiences that shape view of self and other occurred.]

THERAPIST: Is that when it started, do you think? That you would shut down or did you feel comforted by your mom in that moment? ["During a time of need, were you able to rely on a safe other?" is a key question from an attachment point of view.]

RANDY: Oh, she tries to comfort. Yeah, she tried to, you know, to comfort, obviously, but that's when I started to have feelings of fear and anxiety, not being able to explain of course, but just uncomfortable feelings.

THERAPIST: One thing that we find is that when we can stay really still in an experience, it informs us a lot. You're doing a beautiful job of helping me to understand some of that history and some of that experience. And as you talk about it, I'm trying to understand what happens inside your body. Like right now, right here, your eyes, I saw you go for a moment. What happened? I guess you're not sure, maybe, what happened in your body. [Stillness facilitates immediacy. The therapist acknowledges a lack of access versus willingness.]

RANDY: Well, it just makes me feel anxious. Yes, I feel anxious. [Move 2 of the Tango.]

THERAPIST: Like a nausea, or a knot or something different?

RANDY: Just, brr.

THERAPIST: Like shaking?

RANDY: Not shaking, I just feel agitated. [As client goes deeper into experience, vigilance for approval and attempts to "get it right" recede as he begins to explore, discover, and share his inner reality.]

THERAPIST: Agitated.

RANDY: Yeah.

THERAPIST: Or jittery?

RANDY: Jittery? It's something that I don't like, it takes me to places where I feel very uncomfortable. It's very . . . it feels a lot better just kind of, you know . . . [Notice that as the client stays still in experience, experience shifts and clarity deepens.]

THERAPIST: Kind of running around it?

RANDY: Yeah.

THERAPIST: Yeah. I understand. I hear you, Randy. And again, it made perfect sense that that's what you would do. I only partly understand that image, but the picture I have is that your poor mom was probably doing everything she could, but a lot of her resources were elsewhere, so that's part of your alone, is that right?

RANDY: Yes, yeah.

THERAPIST: And the sensation that you have, the feeling that you have in your body, is agitated and jittery? [Therapist reflects and repeats to distill, Move 2 of the Tango.]

RANDY: Yeah.

THERAPIST: So, if we stay really still in it, can we do that? Like, I hear you, of course you want to run from it, but if we try to stay with it, would that be okay? Could you try to stay with it and see what we can discover? [Again, therapist is explicit in saying that we are in a process of discovery. The goal is to keep clients at their leading edge of discovery.]

RANDY: Sure, yeah.

THERAPIST: Because part of the reason that I ask about this, is the more that you can know your automatic experience, the more that you can have flexibility with it. [Collaborative process, therapist provides transparency.]

RANDY: Ahhh.

THERAPIST: And the more that you can have flexibility with revealing to the people that you care about, that you love, that you know you can trust in your brain. But your body's still that little 3-year-old outside. Of course he is, of course. So, if we stay really super still . . . [Therapist remains focused and continues to provide the rationale for the interventions.]

RANDY: Okay, yeah.

THERAPIST: If it's okay.

RANDY: Yeah, it's okay, it's okay.

THERAPIST: What happens to the jitteriness when I invite you to do that? When I slow you down and when you breathe, what happens inside of your body? [Clients often hold their breath, as they did as young children; breathing provides an opening to experience.]

RANDY: Well, it makes me feel, I feel anxiety. It's certainly not comfortable and pleasant, and it just reminds me of not having any control over anything. [Lack of control is a common experience among those who have endured developmental trauma and a poignant reminder of the importance of providing agency in the therapeutic process, ensuring that the interventions are being done "with" the client, not "to" the client.]

THERAPIST: Yeah, scary.

RANDY: Yeah, and that feeling. That's only one teeny weeny little event over a long period of time, but it's the same type of thing that I experienced even yesterday, not feeling in control and feeling not able to defend myself. I'm having to try and protect or . . . it's hard to articulate, it really is.

THERAPIST: That's okay, you're doing a great job. Karen, what's your experience? You're so beautifully holding his hand. What do you feel in these moments, what do you get from his body and from what's happening? [Here the therapist turns to the relationship as a key resource, source of coregulation, as Randy revisits some of this experience, representative of many, and begins to allow himself to feel what he normally "runs" from.]

KAREN: Well, I don't know whether it's him or me, but I can feel a shaking between us, a quivering. I'm not quite sure, maybe it's the coolness. I don't know whether it's the transfer of energy, but I feel kind of cool. I notice that he's not settling into that, he's trying to resist as much as he can, getting to that place. He's not settling into it at all. [Signs of empathy and attunement are a positive indicator for the therapist and for Randy that he is not alone.]

THERAPIST: Have you settled into it?

RANDY: Oh yeah, yeah, I have.

THERAPIST: Okay, okay, okay good, so you have gone into that space.

RANDY: I have.

THERAPIST: In a deep way. Okay.

RANDY: Yeah.

THERAPIST: Okay, maybe you're not comfortable to do it with me, or in this context? [The hesitancy to stay still, to deepen the experience, is explored, space is made for the hesitancy, often referred to as "resistance."]

RANDY: Well, it's very unpleasant.

THERAPIST: Yeah.

RANDY: It's very unpleasant and it's very emotionally draining. It's ugly so no, I don't want to . . . it's not a nice place to go, right?

THERAPIST: Yeah.

KAREN: I think also that when he goes there, he loses control. He's trying, I think desperately right now, to maintain some control, right? Over your emotions?

RANDY: Yeah, yeah, I'm trying to, yeah.

KAREN: I'm just trying to give you some courage.

RANDY: You're staring at me.

THERAPIST: Yeah, I was just thinking about wanting to be respectful, actually, and aware that I'm a new person and this is a new context. I'm wondering how much you would be okay with me helping to contain and to develop and work with this? I get that the resistance is a part of it, that's just a normal thing that happens. I want to be respectful of the role of resistance. [As therapist maintains focus in Move 2 of the Tango, it is with the aim of containing, developing, and deepening experience.]

RANDY: Yes. I think I've come to realize that it's the only way that I'm going to get better.

THERAPIST: True, you're right.

RANDY: I've learned that.

THERAPIST: Okay.

RANDY: But going there is hard, you just don't go there on command, you know? There's just a lot of things, everything, a lot of it's involuntarily, you know? I'm subconsciously going, "Okay, now I'm going to act this way or that way." This is why it's so hard, because it just happens.

THERAPIST: Yes, I know, exactly.

RANDY: It's as natural as breathing, you know?

THERAPIST: Yeah, exactly. And again, that is what happens with kids who have come from difficult home environments. The sort of primitive part of our brains that take care of our basic functions takes over. That's right, it all becomes automatic. [Validation, the EFT form of psychoeducation, and an avenue for providing transparency and agency.]

RANDY: Yeah.

THERAPIST: And we react, and then we realize we reacted.

RANDY: Yeah.

THERAPIST: Or we go into that place, that hole, and then we realize we're there, and wanting to climb out is as scary as all kinds of other things.

RANDY: Yeah.

THERAPIST: So, it all makes sense.

RANDY: Yeah, yeah, that's nice to hear because I didn't think that. A long time ago, with the therapy, I started to realize that, and it gave me a little bit of hope that it's not like I was born this way, you know? [Therapist hears, "It's not me," that there is some part of Randy who knows it was not his fault, but a big part of him that continues to believe that if all these bad things happened, and if he did all these bad things, then he must be bad, unworthy, unlovable.]

THERAPIST: No, absolutely not.

RANDY: So that gave me hope. Sometimes when I think about it, I'm not sure where to go. I'm just talking about what comes to my mind, you know, when I'm talking about my childhood. It didn't have to be that way, you know? [Here again, loss emerges. Therapist maintains focus on immediate goal, to deepen experience; Move 2 of the Tango.]

THERAPIST: Randy, what do you feel when you see that little kid, when you see an image of the little kid? Do you see his little face? [Therapist returns to image to evoke emotion/experience, access self, and ideally, engender some sense of compassion, the antidote to shame, and way forward for increased access.]

RANDY: I feel sad for him, I feel sad.

THERAPIST: Yeah. Can you share that part with Karen? Can you share about the sadness around him and all the loss, and all that he missed out on? Are you able to share that with Karen? [Using Move 3 to resource the client and deepen emotion. Sadness and loss are acknowledged.]

RANDY: Yeah, yeah. Gosh, it's hard sometimes, but I know, Karen, that I go blank, I just go blank. I feel like if it was different, I would be confident.

THERAPIST: Randy, how about this? Can you share that part with her? "When I see that little kid in mommy's arms, the thing that comes up inside of my body is . . . " Can you share that part with Karen? Can you share the feelings that you experience when you see those images? [Deepen, Distill, and Direct; Choreographing the Move 3 encounter.]

RANDY: It's funny, I see a different image now. I see the image, I don't know what time, but I see the image where my mother's crying, and my father's running around and angry, and we retreated to the bedroom. I'm trying to help her, but I can't, I can't, I don't want to go there, and she's crying, and I'm frightened, too. [As is common with trauma, as clients open one doorway to experience, others emerge. Various process elements also are noted, most notably emotion in his voice. The therapist maintains focus.]

THERAPIST: Randy, this is a good place to stay. Can you keep sharing with her what you experience emotionally. If your eyes could speak to her, what would they say? [Move 3 of the Tango: Therapist guides client to keep it visceral, share from body/felt experience.]

RANDY: I don't know, I just feel helpless. I was helpless. I was afraid. She was crying. I'm just there with her. I just felt totally helpless. [Once again, notice how the body provides a gateway to emotion and to felt experience, stillness facilitates immediacy, and as therapist and client maintain focus, emotion/experience deepens and shifts.]

THERAPIST: What happens when you breathe, right now, in your throat? What happens?

RANDY: Uhm, I know I'm pulling back on that emotion because I just about lost it back there. It felt awful. It felt like I couldn't do anything. I was helpless and I wanted to make that go away. I couldn't protect my mother. I couldn't stop my father. I was afraid of him. [Therapist hears exasperation in his voice, fear, terror, and desperation, and notes tear-filled eyes.]

THERAPIST: Karen, in the moment when he shared his tears and he said, "I almost lost it," what happened for you in that moment? [Move 4 of the Tango.]

KAREN: I was feeling that sort of crescendo of emotions as he was, you know, getting to that place, when he's talking about his helplessness. But when he came back and said, "I've pulled back," I can feel that. [Again, a powerful demonstration of attunement. He is not alone.]

THERAPIST: What happens for you, relationally, when he comes in and out of that? In the moment when he was sharing, did you feel like you had him? [Therapist highlights relational impact of tuning in and sharing his felt experience, albeit briefly. Focus is on connection versus pulling back.]

KAREN: Yeah.

THERAPIST: Is that the moment where you feel like he's through the crack? (*Nods yes.*) Have you shared that with him? And what that's like for you? [Move 4 of the Tango, highlighting the impact.]

KAREN: Ah, I don't think so, have I? (*Looking at Randy.*)

THERAPIST: It'd be good for you to share it?

KAREN: Yeah, yeah. So, when you're feeling that way and you're sharing that pain, I feel that with you and I don't want you to be alone. I know I can't go back there, but I'm here with you now and you're not alone. You can tell me and I won't lose my respect for you. I'm sad with you, too. Did your mom know that you were in the room? [Karen explicitly reassures Randy she won't lose respect, and that he is not alone, key ingredients for a corrective experience: "I am with you and accept you."]

RANDY: I was with her when she cried.

KAREN: But did she know you were there with her?

RANDY: Yes.

THERAPIST: To back it up for a moment and sort of focus it on that beautiful moment that you guys just shared, then we can come back to that. So, what she said is that when you risked allowing yourself to open up more and share that feeling—and she could feel it, that's what she was describing—that's when she feels like she can see you and feel you and hear you through the crack, through the armour, right? That would have protected you in all those moments, at times when you couldn't protect your mom. She couldn't protect you and you couldn't protect yourself, yeah? [Therapist maintains focus.]

RANDY: I felt a warmness; I did feel a connection. I did feel something in that time that I've never felt before. [Bodily felt shift is noted.]

KAREN: Is that right?

RANDY: Yes.

THERAPIST: Can you say more about that? If you're able to. Try to stay out of your brain. It's easier to answer the question if you just speak from your gut. [Therapist maintains focus and trusts the wisdom of the body and the power and potency of attachment.]

RANDY: Yeah.

THERAPIST: Or your eyes. What was it? [Again, therapist draws attention to the bodily felt sense, visceral experience—the place where trauma is encoded—and can begin to be transformed. Focus now is on a bottom-up process that can later be cognitively processed and organized.]

RANDY: I just felt warmth and I felt secure. That's something that I never did feel back then at all. [Client explicitly describes a felt sense of security.]

THERAPIST: Did you feel seen? [Therapist maintains focus on restructuring self and system.]

RANDY: Very briefly.

THERAPIST: Yeah, yeah.

RANDY: I've seemed to come back into my shell again, you know?

THERAPIST: You know what, Randy? That's okay, you did amazing. If I can just invite you to stay there for another second?

RANDY: Sure.

THERAPIST: What did you feel like when you felt seen? [Therapist draws attention to impact of tuning in and sharing normally disavowed aspects of self and experience, and of being seen as he did so. Focus is on new experience.]

RANDY: Oh, it is kind of a strange comparison, but it's kind of like where it's a rush of something feeling good. Like when I would escape to alcohol or whatever, I would get a quick rush and that was a really good feeling. But this came from the right place.

THERAPIST: Randy, that's so beautiful. And what I heard you say is that you felt a new experience.

RANDY: Yes, that was a new experience.

THERAPIST: Randy, this is perfect. You come in and out of there as you wish. This is perfect.

RANDY: Yeah, I felt the pain, I felt the ugliness. But in that experience, I just got a tiny glimpse of you being there, your love. A tiny crack, yes. I've never felt that little rush, I'm sorry.

KAREN: I rushed over it really quickly because I was exposing those . . . moments for you, so I'm sorry for changing the subject.

RANDY: It's okay.

THERAPIST: You know what, this is perfect, Randy. You have some flexibility now, right? You can come in and out with her, right here, right now, as you wish. It's kind of like you're peeking from behind your wall and allowing yourself to be seen. Then you can hide again, and she actually doesn't go anywhere. [The momentum of the process, and the session, has now taken hold, giving Randy the flexibility and agency/control he never had as a small child, and the opportunity for connection the couple has been seeking.]

RANDY: No, she's still there.

THERAPIST: It's okay, she knows. It's how it has to be and that's okay.

RANDY: I'm lost for words. I just feel comfortable, and it feels good right now, the . . . anxiety that I was talking to you about. I just feel nice right now.

KAREN: That's good.

THERAPIST: Randy, that's perfect. If you breathe and just stay in your body for a second, deep down, the place you were earlier, what do you feel? [Therapist guides client to stay as long as possible, and as deep as possible, in the experience.]

RANDY: I feel calm and safe. I'm starting to feel relaxed, and I don't want to let go of that nice spot I'm in right now.

THERAPIST: Karen, what do your eyes want to say to him? [Therapist maintains focus on keeping client in experience and sharing it relationally.]

KAREN: It's a place that I've really wanted to go to for a long time, but we disguise things with anger. It's hard because when you react in anger, then I'm provoked to react that way as well, instead of giving you what you really need, which is some empathy and some company. [Karen is contrasting old with new, the therapist will reflect and maintain attention and focus on the new with the aim of keeping the couple and both partners individually at their leading edge.]

THERAPIST: Karen, that's okay, this is good. I get it, this is a whole lot different than that old cycle that you two have been stuck in at times over the years. In your body now, when he shares so beautifully and he is kind of coming in and out, and he is staying still with you, what happens inside your body? I get it, you feel bad about other stuff, but right now, here?

KAREN: Right now, there's a real sense of relief and a real sense of calm. I feel a connection, I think, too, and a warmth. Where before I was, like, trembling because I felt cold, I feel like a real warmth from you, as well. I feel a connection.

RANDY: And I'm holding on because it's just feeling so warm and safe, and it's so different than what I felt yesterday and this morning. If I could feel this way all the time, that'd be beautiful.

THERAPIST: Randy, that's perfect, that's good.

RANDY: Yeah, it feels good, Karen, and I'm not even feeling that anxiety. I don't care about how I was feeling about being insecure and not being good enough. [Therapist maintains focus, is attentive to shifts in view of self and experience, as well as the relationship bond.]

THERAPIST: You feel good enough? [Therapist maintains focus on restructuring self.]

RANDY: In this moment, yes.

THERAPIST: That's so good.

RANDY: Yeah, I'm grabbing on and I'm not letting it go!

THERAPIST: That's good, Randy, that's nice. Is there a word? You said "calm," I think, and "peace."

RANDY: Yeah, I'm not worried or feeling "not enough" at all. I'm not even going there and that is so different than last night. [View of self is changing.]

THERAPIST: That's so good.

RANDY: I'm wondering if it ever felt like this before, growing up, or in my teens, or at any time. I don't want to get into my head but . . . [Therapist hears this as disorientation. Randy is struggling to make sense of and integrate this new experience.]

THERAPIST: No, this is good, Randy, it's perfect. You wanted to ask her?

RANDY: Like, is this how it could be when you're growing up, as you grew up as a kid and as a teenager, as an adult. Is this how you would feel with your parents or your mother or your father? Would you feel safe and comfortable, like what we're experiencing right now? [As Randy speaks and makes contact with his loss and grief, the emotion in his voice and body deepens. He begins to breathe deeply, to sob and heave.]

THERAPIST: There's lots to grieve. It's good to do that, it's good to grieve, that's part of it. She hears you. She's here with you.

RANDY: It hurts so bad.

THERAPIST: That's good, let yourself cry, Randy. It will be good. You'll feel so much better. [The goal is not catharsis, but to encourage Randy to feel what was unsafe and intolerable to feel, literally, in the hands of a safe other.]

RANDY: I didn't know that. I don't know that. I don't know that. [Again, referencing the newness of this experience.]

THERAPIST: It's good if you let yourself breathe and cry. It'll be good, you'll feel better. I'll breathe with you. [The therapist encourages full release, as much as is possible/tolerable, to assist Randy in gaining some sense of liberation from the impacts trauma has had on him, and to fully embrace the sense that he is worthy of love and attention, and very much worth grieving for.]

KAREN: You know how the grandkids come, and they crawl up on your lap, and they snuggle in, and they feel so comforted, you know? They talk to you and are happy to see you. You give that, you give that. [Karen paints a beautiful image of how it should be and was not, and of Randy's resilience to provide what he did not have.]

THERAPIST: Yeah, that's so nice.

KAREN: But you never got it.

RANDY: When you say that, it makes me so sad.

THERAPIST: Exactly, yeah, yeah that's right, Randy, that's true. There's lots to be sad about, for that little boy, right, and what you missed out on. Yeah, it's good. That will be a part of this, to grieve all that.

RANDY: I feel so sad and so good.

KAREN: I feel sad, too.

RANDY: I can't imagine living this way, I can't.

KAREN: You mean the way you live now?

RANDY: No, going through the journey of everything I went through and knowing that . . .

KAREN: It could have been another way.

RANDY: It seems so strange.

THERAPIST: Hmm. You're trying to make sense of all this, yeah?

RANDY: There were so many times when I was so hurt, so alone. Nowhere to go.

THERAPIST: Randy, I can see and feel that now you're trying to kind of make sense of all this, right, and reflecting? But what are you feeling, in your body? [Therapist maintains focus.]

RANDY: I thought I would be feeling anger, you know, but I'm not right now. I'm still feeling good. (*Gazing at Karen and holding her hands tightly.*) I'm feeling your warmth and connection, and I don't want to go away from it. When I think of it, it just makes me so sad.

THERAPIST: Randy, it's good to be sad for him, to be sad for you, it's the right thing, to grieve the loss. And to hear what your beautiful wife is sharing about the grandbabies. It's good that you see the contrast between their little lives and your own.

RANDY: Oh, that breaks me up. How could you treat a little kid bad, how could you do that? (*Sobbing and heaving but with a tone of deep anger now in his voice, assertion.*)

THERAPIST: Exactly, you are right.

RANDY: How could you do that?

THERAPIST: You are absolutely right. [Therapist reinforces contact with need to be loved and accepted, and assertion of needs. Randy conveys contact with a sense of entitlement, of deserving—additional signs of a shifting view of self.]

RANDY: They're so precious. It's just so wrong, it's so wrong. [Therapist hears shift in view of shame, dissolution of shame, "It was wrong/bad, I am not wrong/bad."]

THERAPIST: It is so wrong.

RANDY: Those little kids, they're so perfect, and they don't have to experience what I did. They need to be loved and looked after. They're just so precious.

THERAPIST: Breathe. I think we're all not breathing. You are doing amazing, both of you are so beautiful. Randy, I hear you when you say, "I don't ever want to let this moment go."

RANDY: I don't want to.

THERAPIST: And you know what? You don't actually have to. It's what I said before, that when you . . . well, you tell me when you're ready.

RANDY: I'm ready.

THERAPIST: Are you sure?

RANDY: Yeah.

THERAPIST: I want to give you space, but I'm also aware that it's exhausting, right? Are you okay?

RANDY: I'm okay. I feel comfort and I feel some strength. I feel love, just more safe and loved, and I need it, I need it.

THERAPIST: And you deserve it, absolutely, you deserve it. And you're taking it in which is so good, and in doing so, it puts you right back in touch with the sense of loss that, of course you would feel, in terms of what you didn't have as a little kid. Then you vacillate between cherishing this moment and wanting to hold onto it, but then knowing also what's been missing, right? That's kind of the back and forth you're doing. [Therapist reflects present process and reinforces that he is worthy and deserving.]

RANDY: Yeah.

THERAPIST: Yeah, yeah. It's okay.

RANDY: I feel so good, Karen. It feels good, it really feels good.

KAREN: It's okay.

THERAPIST: Yeah, it's good.

RANDY: I feel so good. I've never experienced this before. It makes me so sad, like, why did it have to be that way? I'm just holding on to you. [Speaking to Karen and continuing to hold her hands, Randy stays with and moves through the experience, the experience he was unable/unsafe to feel at earlier times and shares that with a safe other, trauma is transformed, shame is dissolved, and the bond between the couple deepens and shifts toward secure attachment.]

KAREN: Mm-hmm.

RANDY: And everything that you're giving me right now, no one loved me like that before.

THERAPIST: You're letting her hold you, yeah? (*Nods yes.*) Good. What are you feeling, Karen?

KAREN: Uhm, I feel his pain, but there's also a sensation of being needed.

THERAPIST: Yeah.

KAREN: And so that gives me strength.

THERAPIST: That he'll let you hold him.

KAREN: Yeah.

THERAPIST: Are you okay, Randy?

RANDY: I love it when you do that. I love that, I love this. [Continuing to fully engage with Karen.]

THERAPIST: Yeah, that's good. You know what, Randy? It's back to what I was saying earlier, that when you find your way there, then you have flexibility, more flexibility. It's not going to be perfect, but do you see what happened? Do you see what you did, how you got there earlier? Karen, do you remember? [Introduction to Move 5 summary of the session, moving toward closure and to consolidation and integration of the personal and relational therapeutic gains.]

KAREN: Yeah.

THERAPIST: Yeah. Karen said, "Occasionally, I see that hole, that whatever it is, a teeny bit porous at times, and I can get glimpses of you. I can get glimpses of him." And what you did today, Randy, is that you took the risk of not just taking a glimpse and then going back, but you actually took a real leap of faith and allowed yourself to be seen and felt and heard. And in so doing, you felt a kind of love and security and support that you said you'd never felt before, right? (*Nods and replies, "Yeah."*) And while that's beautiful and amazing, it also brings you right back in touch with what wasn't, and what hasn't been, and there's lots of grieving to do around that. That's where you guys are now, right? Vacillating between these two things. It'll be okay, you'll come up for air. Over the next, you know, week or two, for sure over the weekend. As much as you can live in this space, it'll help you through it, and it's going to be profound. I think it already is, right? And it'll be sustainable. [Move 5 of the Tango.] Does that make sense? (*They both nod.*) And what Karen says is that, in those times, not only does she feel needed. In those moments, Karen, do you feel like you have more than a little glimpse of him? [Therapist highlights and encourages integration, consolidation, and celebration of change, while also inviting the couple to keep the encounter alive.]

KAREN: Oh, absolutely. Yeah, he's all there. [Therapist hears Karen describe a full view of her partner. The authentic self, once eclipsed by shame, was accessed and revealed, leaving Randy feeling seen, heard, and cared for with compassion, and Karen feeling needed in a new way, but also more connected and less alone.]

THERAPIST: And that's part of what she's been fighting for and struggling for, and patiently there waiting for, right? And the more that you risked revealing yourself and sharing with her, the more special she felt. What a gift you just gave her. You said, "I've never, ever, ever, ever, ever felt this way in my life." You risked with her, and she was there, so that's a beautiful treasure that you guys have and share and have worked toward. [Still encouraging the couple to stay in the experience as they are able, therapist uses repetition to evoke emotion.]

RANDY: Yeah, you just break me up when you said, "never experienced before," and I never have. But when you say that, it just evokes so many emotions.

THERAPIST: Yeah, it's okay, you guys did amazing, beautiful, a gift for all of us. Is this a good place to give you guys some space?

KAREN: Sure, yeah.

THERAPIST: Are you okay?

RANDY: I am okay.

Now in the Stage 2 process, next steps for Randy and Karen involved further dissolution of the shame Randy carried, making way for Karen to begin to risk sharing the pain and injury she had endured in the relationship, and for Randy to begin to meet Karen in her pain (see also the attachment injury repair literature, for example, Halchuk et al., 2010; Makinen & Johnson, 2006; Zuccarini et al., 2013). As they were both able to do so, relational attachment wounds were healed, allowing for a further dissolution of Randy's shame, and increased space in the relationship for the acknowledgment and expression of Karen's needs, fears, and longings (see also the pursuer softening literature, such as Bradley & Furrow, 2004, 2007; Myung et al., 2022). As Karen and Randy co-created space and safety for her needs, fears, and longings, and Karen expressed them directly and coherently, this further solidified Randy's view of himself as competent and capable and bolstered his position in the relationship. In turn, Karen's view of herself as special, lovable, and desirable solidified, and their new dance allowed Karen to take a different role in the relationship, that is, less of a caregiver and more of an equal partner.

This might have looked similar in individual therapy. As highlighted in the example featuring Sandy, and in the chapter delineating Sierra's therapeutic work, the main difference centers around Move 3 of the Tango, and the availability of a committed partner. From an EFT perspective, as noted above, change happens in relationship. As such, whenever a physical relationship is available, therapist and client consider the merit of either combining individual and couple therapy, most typically with two separate therapists, or engaging only in couple therapy. In either case, of course, partners can be key resources in harnessing the relationship, in dissolving shame as access to self and experience expands, and in shifting narratives from helplessness to agency, self-sufficiency to reliance, and self-blame and loathing to self-compassion.

PLAY AND PRACTICE

For You Personally

We are all vulnerable to experiences of guilt, regret, embarrassment (i.e., variations of shame). In fortunate circumstances, such experiences are not allowed to fester and impact our ever-evolving self but are instead readily repaired or somehow reconciled with a more prevailing and positive view of self. Can you recall a specific instance of any such experience? How did you find your way out? Or did you (either partially or fully)? If there are lingering impacts from such experiences, how might you address them? What might you do?

For You Professionally

Often in our profession, shame is considered as among the most pernicious and treatment resistant impacts of trauma. If you are new to this work, specifically working with trauma, how might you explain the EFIT approach to working with shame to a colleague or peer also new to trauma work? If you are experienced, are there specific ways you might integrate what you have learned here into your work? What ways? How would you describe this to a colleague or peer?

KEY TAKEAWAYS

Understanding Shame through an Attachment Lens

Shame is an inhibitor—it blocks connection, to self and others.
Shame is adaptive in certain circumstances.
Shame colors the sense of self as bad.
Early cumulative experiences of shame thwart development.

Ways Out of Shame

Repair (see also Attachment Injury Resolution Model)
Meaningful information that challenges shame and associated self-view:

- Strengths
- Positive attachment relationships that can impact and successfully challenge a prevailing negative self-view

▣ New corrective emotional experiences, especially impactful are those choreographed at deep levels

Key Assumptions for Treating Shame in EFT

Shame is relational. Change happens in relationship.
Proximity to self offers a starting point and can be a gauge of progress.
Emotion links self and experience.
Stillness facilitates immediacy.
Shame is contextualized in Stage 1 and more directly addressed in Stage 2.
Compassion is the antidote.
As access and capacity to embody self and experience expands, shame dissolves, and prototypical responses shift from rigidity to flexibility.
Grief naturally emerges as clients gain access to the profound sense of loss that so inevitably accompanies trauma.

Central Differences and Similarities in EFCT and EFIT

Move 3 encounters are choreographed with partners in couple therapy versus imaginal others in individual therapy.
Partners can be resources for one another, but especially in Stage 2 couple therapy.
Social resources are also mobilized, though, in individual therapy, often imaginal initially, then later in therapy, more explicitly highlighted as central to ongoing change.

8

Consolidation in Stage 3

Turning now to the final stage of therapy, Stage 3, Consolidation, we again draw attention to the four CARE dimensions and the key roles of each in supporting the client in continuing to consolidate, integrate, and build on therapeutic gains. Contextual factors are considered in highlighting risk and protective factors, and attention is drawn to the client's increased flexibility and capacity, and the ongoing ability to employ longstanding coping/protective strategies if/and as needed. Central characters in the client's story are called upon to provide their perspective on therapeutic progress, and to support continued growth. Shifts in the client's narrative are illuminated. A vision for the future, needs, goals, and aspirations are highlighted. A new narrative that integrates the past and holds hope for the future is shaped. Shifts in model of self are exemplified, consolidated, and integrated. New action tendencies and increased flexibility are made vivid, highlighting a wider gap between trigger and response, and offering a broader repertoire of behavioral responses (action tendencies). New ways of being and belonging are highlighted and celebrated. Sensitive attunement guides the structuring of final sessions, possibly in anticipation of major life events and/or anniversaries, or perhaps, on a more regular but infrequent basis, again, depending on various factors such as context.

Introducing another generous and inspiring client, Yezda, this chapter provides a summary of the first session, along with a transcript from a Stage 3 session, to highlight the attachment-focused clinical picture at the outset of therapy, and compare it with that in later sessions, particularly in Stage 3 of the three-stage EFT process. As is the case in Stages 1 and 2, clients most typically engage in more than one session in Stage 3, but with the organic growth process unleashed and the momentum of the process taken hold outside the therapy process, sessions are often less frequent. Secure attachment remains the therapist's beacon and guiding light, as characterized by the capacity to tune into one's internal world—needs, fears, longings, vulnerabilities—share those coherently and directly with a key trusted other, and give and receive care and love. In Stage 3, with more ready access to model of self, the therapist has the opportunity to not only gauge and consolidate gains, but in so doing, also continue to restructure and reshape attachment. Inquiries are made with attention to view of self and system, as well as affect regulation strategy and capacity.

Although the focus and target of change remains the heart of the matter, specifically attachment security, attention is also drawn to shifts in the more surface-based symptom picture that, of course, is relevant, and especially when clients present for therapy with concerns about symptoms at the forefront. Symptom resurgences are anticipated as likely (e.g., in the context of exposure to new trauma, trauma-related cues and/or anniversaries of key events such as trauma or loss) and are not suggestive of setbacks but are instead indications of ongoing vulnerability, now diminished with increased capacity, and with the ability to reach for and receive support. In short, just as secure attachment affords couples the opportunity to more readily and effectively repair following conflict, so too is it expected that individuals will more easily and successfully regain their emotional balance in times of stress or distress. Secure attachment leads to increased resilience.

When clients can come home to themselves, to their inner emotional worlds, and their previously disavowed or disowned aspects of self and experience, the outcome is a more integrated, confident, competent sense of self. The natural progression is the navigation and/or renegotiation of relationships with key others. As clients gain compassion for themselves, they often also gain compassion for others. With increased capacity to tune in and trust their internal experience and use it as a compass for life and love, the therapist does not guide or prescribe relations with others but instead trusts, supports, and celebrates the internal wisdom of each client. At times, the renegotiation of relationships involves giving up hope that a loved one can ever provide the acceptance, care, and love that the individual now recognizes was deserved but not provided. When the impacts of trauma are disentangled from self and story, and when trauma is transformed and clients find their agency, perception will broaden and choice deepen, leading to decisions that best suit the needs of the client. Recognizing the value of grief in providing space for something or someone new, the therapist supports this central aspect of the process. As with symptoms, it can be expected that grief might emerge as an anticipated (e.g., at anniversaries or birthdays) and unexpected guest at various times in the client's life. Clients are encouraged to welcome and embrace such experiences, rather than downplaying or dismissing them, honoring self and experience, and continuing to make space for something or someone new.

At the beginning of Session 1, Yezda tells the therapist that she feels the need to seek therapy as she anticipates her upcoming wedding, just weeks away. She recognizes that her efforts to forget her past are impacting her future. She is afraid to have a family, fearful she might exhibit some of her parents' "traits," or be triggered by them. She does not know who she is, and she is unclear about her capacity to somehow make sense of the rich cultural history her parents brought to Canada. With her mother from South America and her father a war refugee from Iraq, Yezda has some sense of the worlds they grew up in, but not fully. Her father's family was "land rich" and her paternal grandfather was in her father's words, "Chief of his tribe." She is aware he beat her grandmother but is uncertain whether he also abused his other wives. Conscripted to fight in a war that would involve killing his own people, Yezda's father fled Iraq and taught English in other countries before moving to Canada in his 20s. Her mother grew up in poverty, left school when she was 9 or 10 years old, and was sent to Canada to live with relatives, and in later years was commanded to remain to build a life and to bring her family to Canada. This is what she did.

In sharing her parents' histories, Yezda explained, "I've heard the stories many times, it feels like I'm talking about a movie, it doesn't feel like my life." She has worked hard to separate herself from those stories, especially because her mother began to share these and other accounts of domestic violence when Yezda was very young with the motive, she conjectured, to evoke sympathy and an allegiance with her daughter. Yezda became her mother's confidante and protector, "a shield" from her father's abuse during their frequent fights.

Continuing to recount her childhood during that initial session, her fine facial features mostly still and her eyes locked straight ahead, Yezda seemed to carefully choose her words. She appeared stoic. She was articulate. Further describing her own relationship with her parents, she recalled good memories with her dad, learning to ride a bike and to rollerblade, walks in the neighborhood punctuated with breaks to share cut fruit. "I remember warmth from him," she said, in contrast to the anxiety she felt in the presence of her mother, describing a sense of being controlled, of unpredictability, and of fear. "I still sometimes have this lump in my throat that creeps up that reminds me of when my dad would go to work, and I'd be left at home with my mom."

In recounting various key events in childhood, Yezda referenced memories of vomiting in her mother's arms as her mother fled her husband's wrath, then being left downstairs until her mother returned.

At age four, her father changed her name to better represent his own cultural identity. When asked about her parents' names and places of birth for her wedding license, Yezda struggled. They both changed their names when they came to Canada, and neither parent was aware of their place of birth. "Something that is so easy for a lot of people is often really challenging for me and this is just one of the things that is starting to come up for me this year."

She recalled learning to read *The Night Before Christmas* in December, her mother slapping her each time she made a mistake, and her baby sister crying as she sat on her mother's lap. She was in grade one. "She would tell me that I was stupid and that the other kids would laugh at me if they knew I couldn't read." Yezda conveyed that her mother wanted to protect her from being teased or discriminated against, as she herself had experienced.

As she got older, her mother also wanted to prevent any "unwanted attention" from boys in the community. She did not let Yezda cut her hair. She controlled the clothes Yezda wore, and did not allow Yezda to shave her legs. "I grew up in a really white community and I was one of the few minorities at my school. I didn't want to stand out in that way and my parents also didn't want us to stand out. I think that's why we didn't practice a lot of cultural things at home, because they didn't want us to. They wanted us to be Canadian; although if my dad talks about it now, he talks about being Canadian in a negative way, and he's disappointed that I'm marrying a Canadian, especially one who is not Muslim."

Despite her parents' efforts to hide aspects of their culture and history so they wouldn't "stand out," be discriminated against, or harmed in any way, Yezda was bullied in school. She often felt misunderstood or wholly dismissed. Yezda did not feel any sense of belonging, either at home or at school.

Now some years later, she described the conflict between seeking a sense of belonging and holding onto her cultural identity. "I feel like so much of my life has been wanting to be different and blend in and to feel like I am at the same level as others who were born in this country. But then I'm being pulled back in a different way and sitting in this space where I don't really know my cultural identity that well because my parents separated us from it. I don't really know where I am with that."

According to Yezda, the children never experienced any direct abuse from their father, and it all stopped between their parents when she was in mid-adolescence, following successful treatment of her father's "chemical imbalance" with the introduction of medication. Also, during that time, she established some autonomy through working at a coffee shop and earning her own money. Even then, however, she felt her mother continued to sabotage her efforts for success in dancing (a key source of competence and refuge). Physical and emotional abuse from her mother also were ongoing, including threats and incidents of assault with weapons, such as wooden spoons, umbrellas, and broom handles.

"God and Allah were present in their home," more like a "cultural observing" than a practicing of faith, she explained, though she spent many hours praying to God that she would find her way out of the life she had been born into. Temporary means of escape included watching movies about travel and going to different places. A map adorned her bedroom wall, with pins denoting anticipated destinations, along with photos of universities she planned to attend. The family next door provided a window into "a different way of living," as did a boyfriend in late adolescence.

Four years later, in her early twenties, she met her fiancé. Yezda described it as akin to meeting someone she already knew, an "electric current" pierced through her body. He was different. The relationship was different. He asked questions most people didn't ask. He was curious about her cultural background, rather than assuming she was of Indian descent, as most people had done up to that time. His history of trauma and loss also drew her to him. She felt she could share with him, and he wouldn't be afraid. She described him as "the answer to her letters to God, someone who would save me and understand me."

Now, over 10 years later, her parents continued to live in the same house she grew up in, and though she had left years ago with the hope to forget her past, she continued to be haunted by the many memories she had tried to escape. Dreams of her mother dying continued to interrupt her sleep.

As a child, she would lay awake, vigilant for the possibility her mother might harm herself. Her mother had shared a prior suicide attempt and Yezda felt responsible for preventing another. Her parents slept in separate rooms and Yezda's room was across the hall from her mom's. She would listen for the sound of pills rustling.

Various smells, images, and sounds continue to trigger her, leading to increased anxiety, and reinforcing feelings of being out of control, and unable to prevent the negative impacts of her childhood. Any hint of criticism or blame from her fiancé is also a reminder and sets her back. "I get triggered when my fiancé attempts to provide me with feedback or asks me about my business decisions. I inflate it. I make it bigger than it is. I feel criticized. I get tense—feel tension in my chest. Again, I feel unsupported, alone. I get angry. I try to defend myself and then I shut down. I get quiet and then I usually leave the room." In shutting down, Yezda referenced withdrawal and emotional numbing, though drugs and alcohol had never been contributing factors. She had also never been formally diagnosed, though she had engaged in therapy at various times.

In looking back on the landscape of her life, Yezda described an image of a young child, alone on the elementary school playground, about 6 years old. "She is lonely and tired, and sad and doesn't know why." Initial attempts to make contact are successful, and the young child can take in the comfort of an "older wiser adult Yezda"—a positive indicator of capacity, though an ongoing propensity to avoid was also noted in her statement, "I try to forget that time."

In concluding the initial session, the therapist replied and summarized, providing a road map for therapy: "Yezda, that makes perfect sense—what I hear you saying is how you coped with a really unpredictable home life . . . you said that it was predictable and stable in a lot of ways, your family is still in the same home you grew up in and the community was relatively stable, but in terms of the behaviors and the conflict, the fear of loss and fear of danger, that part was unpredictable. You carried a lot of it as the oldest child and as the confidante and protector to your mom. And then as we transport ourselves to the school ground, you say that little girl is tired and alone. I hear you; there's a part of you that doesn't want to get close to that, but I'm also struck by your capacity to do so and that she was so readily able to accept your accessibility and care. So Yezda, as we work together, the more that you can be in touch with her and allow her to be with you and help her—and I'm going to help you, too, I'm going to be alongside you, too—the more you feel some of the feelings that were not safe to feel as a little girl . . . because it was way better to transport yourself and imagine something else . . . and we don't have to dredge up every memory and work through every event that shaped and characterized those early years, but enough that you have control of them and your emotional reactivity and sensitivity, as you were describing earlier. Then you can be fully grounded in yourself in a different way that allows you to move more deeply and more readily into the vulnerability that wouldn't have been safe to experience in those earlier times. The intent is to offer you choice, agency. The thing I hear you saying is that there were a lot of things taken from you in your childhood, including your cultural history. Now, it makes sense that you have confusion when you think about marriage, developing your own family identity, and having your own children and thinking about how you'd want to raise them, even the questions that come up around names and your parents' places of birth. Of course, all these things are coming back, so this is a good time to move through some of this in a way that gives you more choice, choice that you didn't have as a young person. You do now, and I feel your strength and your clarity and your knowing. This is just going to add to that, Yezda. Does that make sense and fit for you?" "Yeah," she answered, "because I think what I'm realizing is that I don't know how I really felt as that child because I was always trying to not feel. I pushed away from being present."

As we accompany Yezda in exploring key pivotal moments that have shaped her sense of self, various doorways are opened and she is encouraged to begin to feel, in the imaginal company of trusted others, such as her older wiser self and her partner, what was intolerable to feel at the time of various central defining events.

With the same stoicism observed in initial sessions, an encounter with her parents during one of their many arguments leaves her with a newfound sense of agency. Rather than retreating and sheltering her younger brother and sister from the turbulence in their parents' relationship, Yezda boldly stands firmly in the hallway of the family home and silently yells at them both to "Stop!" As she gingerly reveals what just happened, she also describes a tingling in her toes. The quiver in her voice is quiet but audible. The trauma that lives in her body is being awakened as she moves closer to and remains present with her experience.

Additional encounters are similarly aimed at choreographing corrective emotional experiences—moments of contact with herself and her experience in these key relational events that have shaped her—this time, not alone, and each time with an increased capacity to feel what was unsafe to feel as a little girl, as an adolescent, and as a young woman. As the therapeutic process unfolds, so too does Yezda's capacity to feel. Her sense of self similarly begins to expand.

Midway through the process, amid another encounter in the family home, when young Yezda asks her older wiser self, "Why don't I deserve to be loved and protected?" Yezda firmly and confidently replies that she does deserve to be loved and protected. "This is not right. It's not your fault" is a key identity epiphany shaped deep in experience—a redefining change event in therapy.

With the ongoing progression of therapy, Yezda similarly redefines her position as caregiver, protector, and confidante in her family. With increased capacity, during one of the sessions in an imaginal encounter with her mother, she asserts herself with her mother while protecting herself with a shield made of plexiglass. A pivotal shift. Yezda describes feeling "less vulnerable, like the ground beneath me is more solid." She is now able to begin to let go of the vigilance and stoicism that have restricted her and prevented her from playing as a little girl and living fully as an adult.

The grips of her past now loosened, Yezda is beginning to see herself and her relationships in a new light, and her history and future with more clarity. The transcript to follow represents a Stage 3 session with

Yezda, edited for brevity and clarity. Again, therapist commentary is provided.

THERAPIST: Yezda, what's your point of view in terms of where you were when we started together and where you are now? [Therapist begins with an open-ended question and continues to maintain a stance of curiosity and cultural humility.]

YEZDA: I think it depends on the day. I do often feel like sometimes I have one foot in the past and one foot in the future, and I feel very split sometimes. I'm trying to fight to be the person that I envision for myself, while also trying not to discount or shove down what's happened in the past. I've done it for a long time, a lot longer than I thought and in ways I didn't realize. One of the ways I have changed is with respect to who I see myself as now, in terms of culture and background and upbringing, and how it's impacting me as a person now. I definitely feel I have more clarity as to who I am now. I can almost separate what's happened in the past and be able to sit in it and reflect on it more than I was able to and see how it's connected to how things happen with me now. Sometimes I feel in between these two people, but I do see myself sitting more in the person I'm trying to be. That's been freeing in a lot of ways, and as I start to have more contact with my parents, which I have had in the last few weeks, I feel stronger and better able to deal with them, instead of my stomach churning every time I think about calling them or talking to them. [Various indicators of change are noted, most prominently, increased awareness and capacity to understand past and impact on present, as well as improved ability to maintain emotional balance in interactions with parents, two of the key characters who continue to live in her heart and mind.]

THERAPIST: Good for you! That's great Yezda. When you describe two different people and when you look back at you, and connect with your past, who do you see in that picture? [Therapist focuses on self; the key goal in EFIT is to expand the self. The inquiry is aimed at discerning vision of self at outset relative to now.]

YEZDA: I see someone who's lost, someone who doesn't really know who they are and isn't really feeling like they know where to go to find that out. I can remember the early years of moving out of my parents' house and moving in with Sam. I was trying to almost pretend to be someone completely different. I remember having this thought about moving across the country to be with Sam and thinking, "I'm going to be whoever I want to be now," and it felt inauthentic, it felt like I was forcing myself to be a certain person.

THERAPIST: Do you know who that person was?

YEZDA: Yeah, it was a bit of me trying to be like Sam's sister-in-law, Gabriela. She was well-respected and really loved in the family. She was someone who was really independent and didn't rely on anyone.

THERAPIST: Yezda, I'm struck by what you're saying around wanting to emulate somebody who was really loved. Is that what you were hoping for? A sense of belonging and love in that family? [At other times in the therapy process, Yezda has expressed a desire to feel closer to Sam's family, and to feel more accepted.]

YEZDA: I think it was more to do with Sam because I really wanted the relationship to work, especially because I had taken such a, I don't want to say "gamble," but I had taken such a big step around leaving what I had planned for myself and trying the relationship out. I think that was safe for me, in some ways, instead of going out completely on my own. It was a good transition for me. I never really reflect back too much on why I made that decision, other than I saw someone who really wanted to be with me and saw me for who I was, and I was really drawn to that.

THERAPIST: That sounds like it captures what you were looking for, a sense of belonging and love and autonomy, being able to have both, is that right?

YEZDA: I think early in our relationship, it was really challenging because Sam wasn't quite ready to have the relationship that we were imposing on ourselves because we were so young. I think I was judged a lot by him in the beginning, and he often reflected on what he felt like our relationship should be based on his brother's relationship to his wife Gabriela. And that caused a lot of tension, and it took us a while to get over that. I don't feel like we got over it in those early years. I feel like it wasn't until a few years ago that we were able to overcome some of the resentment that came from that, but there were periods of time where I felt more accepted by him than I did with my parents.

THERAPIST: What was it about their relationship that he wanted to emulate?

YEZDA: On the outside, it seemed pretty effortless for them. She really respected him and gave him his space. They just jived well together. They were also very involved in the family too and it was never a sticky area with how involved they were. They were always giving of themselves and their time to the family.

THERAPIST: Oh, I understand, that's really valued in that family, isn't it?

(*She nods in agreement.*) Yezda, when you look at you now, what do you see? [Therapist returns to focus on self.]

YEZDA: I see that we are able to define it for ourselves now. I see that there is respect around who we are in the family and who we are as a couple. We're very far from comparing ourselves now because I think we're happy with where we're at, in terms of how we work together in our relationship. We're not trying to grasp at anyone else's to compare.

THERAPIST: And when you look and see you, who do you see? What do you see? [Therapist maintains focus on direct *assessment* of view of self.]

YEZDA: I think for me, especially in the last few weeks, I'm feeling a lot more relaxed and confident in who I am. I'm not trying to be someone else, and I feel like there's been more energy that's been freed up because I'm more confident and comfortable with who I am now that I'm opening space to do even more personal growth. I feel like I can see myself as that person that I want to step into more clearly now. And with that comes leaving behind that clenching I always felt, or that every move I made was being judged or questioned. I don't feel self-conscious anymore. [Therapist hears that Yezda is more relaxed and confident, not "clenching" in anticipation of judgment, and more comfortable with who she is.]

THERAPIST: Yezda, that's so great. I appreciate your ability to see your progress! So, when you see yourself stepping into you, who do you see? Who is that person? [Therapist maintains focus on view of self as a means of assessing, highlighting, integrating, and consolidating therapeutic gains.]

YEZDA: Someone who will make mistakes but they're not so hard on themselves. I'm looking more inward than I have in the past. I've always looked at who I was and how I affected others, but especially in the last few days, it feels almost vulnerable to be in this space because all these feelings around what I've accepted in the last few years are coming up. For example, yesterday was a challenging day for me. Sam and I had gone out to eat, and twice people had asked if we were together. Those little comments that I used to just glaze over, or I wouldn't acknowledge, now they're hitting me a bit harder because I'm, like, "Why are they asking me that?" It's not normal to ask that, it's not standard. In the past I would say, "Oh maybe that's a default," but I'm always making excuses for other people's bad behaviors.

THERAPIST: Good for you Yezda, now you're seeing you. [Trending toward self-care and protection rather than the care and protection of others, shift in key element of attachment.]

YEZDA: Yes, and I'm acknowledging me. I had this conversation with my coach this morning about what that means to me as a leader because I never felt like I could be just a person in my team. I felt that my feelings weren't as important as everyone else's, so if the team was upset or someone had an issue, I had to put myself aside. I never shared how that affected me. I never felt like that was as important, but I feel like now, that person I'm seeing, that their feelings and their emotions are just as important. I should give space to reflect on that more, instead of just shoving it down. I think with that comes me being kinder to myself too because I put a lot of pressure on myself as well. [Therapist hears growing sense of entitlement—"I am important."]

THERAPIST: "I matter," that's what I hear you saying, "I matter, I'm important here, too. So are my needs, my feelings, and experiences." [Therapist reflects that which we want the client to notice/consolidate.] What I hear you saying is as you step into the person you are—and of course it's all evolving and you're growing, and you're growing in your relationship—the you that's there feels a bit more vulnerable because you're allowing yourself to feel some of what you negated or dismissed at other times in your life. I appreciated what you said, that you were just glossing over your own experience and excusing people for their bad behavior, and now you're actually seeing you and allowing yourself to feel. When you see you in those moments, like in the restaurant, for example, that you were just describing, what do you see when you have that kind of an experience? What do you see on the inside of you? [Therapist invites client to revisit scene and inhabit internal experience.]

YEZDA: More of an acceptance of me. It's going to be hard for me to describe this and I think I've mentioned to you how hard my identity has been for me to digest over the last few years, but for as long as I can remember, I've never considered the color of my skin or my defining cultural features. I didn't know until I was older in life that the way I look separates me in some ways from others, and so in my brain, until recently, I didn't really think about some of the reactions I get and that some of the ways I was treated may be because of that. I'm glad that it didn't hold me back, but I'm starting to see more of myself in the way that I actually am, instead of how I've been perceiving myself in how I think I look like everyone else.

THERAPIST: Yezda, I'm so moved by what you're saying. The thing I hear you saying is, "As I step closer to me, I'm finding myself, my background, my identity in new and different ways, in ways that I didn't recognize." [Key shifts are summarized to promote integration and consolidation.]

YEZDA: I think also, with not being close with my parents and having such a challenging relationship with them, I was embarrassed or ashamed of coming from those backgrounds because I feel like it contributed to the situation. As in, if I had had Canadian parents, maybe I wouldn't have had to witness domestic abuse or violence toward myself. So, I feel like I put myself further away from that and now it's coming up, now that I've married outside of the culture and I'm sitting in it more. I reached out to my parents and said I wanted to get citizenship from their countries.

THERAPIST: From both of their countries?

YEZDA: Yes.

THERAPIST: Yezda that is so great, that is so good!

YEZDA: That was something that I talked to them last week about. So, I'm working through that and I'm really starting to feel like who I am, what I represent, and that where I came from really matters more now.

THERAPIST: Good for you, that is so beautiful! That's part of what I hear you saying, that as you disentangle you and your cultural identity from some of those experiences associated with your history, you can find you in new ways. I think you said it beautifully in a session not long ago, as well. As you move through the more difficult aspects of your childhood and things, I heard you say words like "manipulation" and "control" and "oppression," and it was all mixed together. But now, as you work through some of those felt experiences, you can see and feel and be enriched by this beautiful, rich history that you carry, and that others noticed before you did. Is that capturing it?

YEZDA: Yeah, I think so and I think now I'm not tying my culture and background to my history. Being Kurdish on my dad's side doesn't mean I'm him, it means that that's my history. I'm able to separate that more now for myself.

THERAPIST: Right and when you say "him," you're referring specifically to the aspects of him that were not positive in your relationship.

YEZDA: Yeah.

THERAPIST: I appreciate how you describe "him," even from the beginning Yezda. It still sits with me, the beautiful image. You know what I'm going to say probably, don't you?

YEZDA: The walks with my dad. (*Smiles.*)

THERAPIST: Exactly! And sharing the fruit. Those lovely moments, his tenderness.

YEZDA: Mmmm. (*Smiling.*) Part of the reason why I decided to get Iraqi citizenship was because I knew how special that would be for him.

THERAPIST: Yezda, that's so nice!

YEZDA: I knew that it was a big deal for him to accept me marrying outside of the culture and I know that the stubborn side of me is like, "Well he lives in Canada, he should expect it," but now I understand that so much of my identity is tied to his culture. Yes, I'm proud to be of that cultural background. I want him to know that as well and that I acknowledge it, because I think he's always felt like he's been trying to impose it on us our entire lives. So, for me to come to him and say, "Hey I'm embracing it now," I think is a really big deal for him.

THERAPIST: That's beautiful Yezda, so touching! Do you hear what you're saying? About how far you've come?

YEZDA: Yeah, I think so. I think the biggest thing is that I'm able to see me more and see who I am, and accept and celebrate where I've come from, that it wasn't all bad.

THERAPIST: Beautiful, absolutely beautiful! And how would that look? What does that celebration look like?

YEZDA: I think going through this process of getting citizenship and talking to my dad more about what it means to him. I told him that I had hired someone who had spent time in Turkey, and we had talked about it for a little bit. She, this person I had hired, speaks four different languages and she went to Turkey as a translator. Then it spurred this conversation and he's like, "Well you know I speak seven languages," and I said, "You know I know that." So, we're at this weird place where he's starting to forget how much I know about him because so much time has passed since I've been on my own. But I think it's important for us to have more of those conversations so that he feels like I see him, too. [In a later session, Yezda shared that she was formally interviewing her father to learn more of his story and to document it.]

THERAPIST: Yezda, that's so powerful, isn't it? "I see you, and as I see me, I see more of you," and "It's easier for me to share how much I see and know of you."

YEZDA: It's very draining all of this, going through this process. It's been good, but I have moments where I'm really tired, when I'm reflecting on all the layers and all of what's happened.

THERAPIST: Yes, Yezda, it's important work and you've done so much! We talk in our world about an organic growth process. As we help people make sense of the barriers to that, and the blocks that we can all get caught in in terms of our context, history, and the here and now, there's this ongoing process. You will and you are, going to continue to grow and work through some of those difficult times in your life. You've done a lot of that and now you can see you in new ways and grow you in new ways and assert you in new ways. It really is evident, and it's great! That's part of why, I think, we both talked about this being so important, to punctuate all this amazing work, to look back and into the future in ways that really allow you to see and feel and celebrate you. Fantastic—all the amazing work you've done!

YEZDA: I do feel like I'm less nervous about things creeping up unexpectedly now, too, because I know that was big. When you and I started doing sessions together, a big concern for me was how some of that trauma and past experiences would creep up in different ways for me. I was a bit of a ticking time bomb, where one bad thing could happen at work and . . . I think the loss of control was a really big concern for me. It's not perfect but I think I'm further from feeling like that would happen. [The therapist hears this as the space between trigger and response widening, and the behavioral repertoire also expanding; less automaticity and rigidity.]

THERAPIST: That's wonderful Yezda, that's beautiful. I'm not surprised you say that, but it's great to hear you say it. It helps to clarify where you are. So, when you think about your mom, where are you with your mom? Do you know? [The therapist assumes that as clients come home to themselves, they will use their inner emotional worlds as a compass to navigate and/or renegotiate key relationships in the manner that is best for them, and with the understanding that as they continue to grow and shift, so too, might their most important relationships.]

YEZDA: I am talking to her more, which I think helps and she's trying to cultivate more of a relationship with Sam, which I appreciate. I still feel like she's very manipulative, so when I talk to her, it's not a fully open and vulnerable conversation. I still feel very guarded a lot of the time. I talked to her a couple weeks ago. I don't know what I called about but she automatically defaulted to starting to complain about my dad, and I was really brought back to being young again and sitting in her room and listening. Sometimes it would be hours where she would unload on me about how my dad was, and how much he drove her nuts. So that brought me back a little bit, and that was challenging. In the end she apologized for complaining about him, but I don't know if it was authentic or if she could just read the energy that I wasn't appreciating it because I didn't really engage that much, I just let her speak about it. I don't feel close to her and sometimes I wonder if I will ever feel that way with her and if it's okay that I don't. She still doesn't feel safe to me. One thing with the announcement this week about the light at the end of the tunnel with COVID, is I know that Sam will want to travel home to visit family and then I instantly had a thought like "Oh we can travel now. Oh, we can go visit family" and then my chest instantly tightened up because I was like, "What happens when we go back home? Who do we stay with?" I haven't been home in two and a half years, and the last time I was there, I left my parents' house because my mom and I got into an argument, and I stayed in a hotel until my flight a couple of days later. I've never gone back and not stayed with them, and my reaction, my default, would be to stay with Sam's parents and him. I think it would be too awkward and not appropriate for Sam to stay with me at my parents' house because traditionally what we've done is stayed separately with our own parents. So, I have to work through that now and see what that looks like for me.

THERAPIST: I hear you Yezda. Is that in your picture now? What I understood you to say around this in the past is that you and Sam met when you were really young and your dad had certain expectations, but it sounds like Sam's now accepted, from what you said, and by your mom, too, actually. And what you're saying now is that she's nurturing that relationship with Sam even more, with recipes and cooking tutorials. What would their expectation be? Do you feel you shouldn't stay there together?

YEZDA: I don't think that would be their expectation, especially for my dad. He doesn't ever bring Sam up and he hasn't met Sam officially so I think that staying there together would be too much.

THERAPIST: Right, that would be a lot for your dad all at once. I hear you. Do you imagine what it's going to be like when he meets Sam?

YEZDA: I haven't wrapped my head around that, although I know it'll happen, but I don't sit in it too much because his reaction to telling him really was surprising for me. I know that he knows now and that's the biggest thing, so I don't try to spend too much time and energy worrying about what their first meeting is going to be like. I think it'll probably be awkward but I'm trying to be optimistic! (*Smiling.*)

THERAPIST: How does Sam feel about it?

YEZDA: I think Sam will be fine. Sam is not ignorant of challenging or uncomfortable situations so I feel like he can make the best of it. I think it'll be interesting to see my dad. My brain can't handle that scenario so I think I'm just, like, "Well, we'll see what happens." I told them over the phone about getting married, and then I got married and they weren't there. It's such a weird universe, like, they know but it doesn't feel real just yet because they haven't met.

THERAPIST: Yeah, you know what I reflect back to? Your dad having tea in your home. Do you remember that? In this home, the home you're in now. [This image emerged in an earlier session in therapy, in the context of imagining having a child, the pride he would feel, and the desire he would have to be a part of his grandchild's life.]

YEZDA: Oh yeah, that vision of seeing him here? I think for some reason that's easier for me to think about instead of going home because there's so many other things swirling around, other emotions, other past experiences. Even just being in that house is really hard for me, but if they were to come here, I would be in more control of the situation.

THERAPIST: True, that's a good point.

YEZDA: Yeah, and I'm more myself here. I know who I am here but when I go back, it always feels like a push and pull, that my mom is trying to drag me back to how it was before. So that's the constant battle when going home.

THERAPIST: What does your mom say about you wanting to get citizenship with her country?

YEZDA: I think she was excited, and I think she was surprised. She called me. She had found some info for me and called me. I missed her call. I have to call her back. It's funny because I called them and they didn't say anything about, like, "Oh you have to help your brother and sister do it too," so I was appreciative that they didn't impose that on me.

THERAPIST: Yeah, that's great. Will your brother and sister do that?

YEZDA: I don't know, I think my sister might. It's one of those things where even if they ask me to help, I would tell them that it has to be their decision. I will help and support them but I'm not going to do it for them, which I always do. For my brother and sister, I was always that person to take care of things for them. [Highlighting another change in self and system/relations with key others.]

THERAPIST: Yezda, I am just so impressed and struck by everything you're saying. That sentence, "I am not going to be the caregiver in my family anymore. I'm going to care, and I do care. As I find me, it gets easier to separate myself from them and to appreciate and embrace the aspects of me and my history that I never had the space for at other times." [Again, therapist repeats and reflects to promote further integration and consolidation.]

YEZDA: It's a funny space to be in right now. I was happy that I got the last three weeks, because I felt like I overcame me the last little while. I did feel a release a week ago where I'm, like, "This feels okay. I don't have to worry about anything. I don't have to be a certain way, I don't have to act a certain way, and I don't have to worry about hiding a secret or live up to anyone's expectations."

THERAPIST: What do you feel in your body as you share all this?

YEZDA: It feels like a letting go, which is nice. It feels very freeing for me to know that and actually see what that looks like because I would see it before, but it wouldn't compute in my head as to what that actually meant. It was something I knew I wanted to work toward but didn't know how to do it.

THERAPIST: Do you know how you did it?

YEZDA: I mean, all this work.

THERAPIST: Revisiting some of those scenes and working through them emotionally, and finding compassion for yourself and finding you. Then really beginning to look at your home life and your family life through a different lens, potentially a broader lens.

YEZDA: Yeah, and I think one of the biggest things for me was accepting that what happened did have an impact on me. I think I really refused to think that. I was, like, "Okay, I left my parent's house; I'm not living at home, this is not an issue anymore," but there was more to it than that, and accepting that more. I can remember arguments that Sam and I had five to six years ago where he would be, like, "Why are you reacting like this? Where is this coming from?" And it would make me even more angry, and I'd be like "Nothing, I'm just angry about what's happening right now, it has nothing to do with anything else, there's no underlying cause!" (*Therapist and client both smile.*) [Therapist hears this as creating a new narrative that integrates her story but also liberates her from the hold it had on her, a story that integrates the past and holds hope for the future.] I always wanted to be honest because I always wanted to be better, and I think that's really helped.

THERAPIST: Yezda, you are amazing, so strong and clear. It's really touching to sit with you. It's just such a lovely experience to join you in looking back! When you look forward, what do you see? Just from your body, Yezda, just your body, if your chest, if your throat could speak. What is the vision out there that comes to you, just from your body? [Yezda now has contact with herself and her inner experience in ways she did not have in earlier times and at the outset of therapy. Therapist directs Yezda to her body, the seat of emotion and experience, to guide her in moving forward.]

YEZDA: I think just feeling more grounded was a big one. I'd felt this feeling a lot, that feeling of being grounded was what I was working toward, and it really helped through this process. So, when I think about it, or what I feel in my body, it's me feeling lighter, but my feet are more planted. [Therapist hears this as a direct comparison to one of the initial sessions aimed at helping Yezda begin to contact and feel frightening, alien, and unacceptable emotion.]

THERAPIST: Yezda, isn't that amazing? "I feel lighter, but my feet are more planted." That is very poignant. "I feel lighter, but my feet are more planted." And when you look at that little girl on the playground what do you see? [Therapist refers to the scene and vision of self from Session 1 as a means of gauging progress, as well as highlighting, consolidating, integrating, and celebrating gains. Once again, assessment and treatment merge.]

YEZDA: I see her looking over at me, and she's kind of curious. She wants to know what's going on and almost doesn't recognize the person that she's looking at, but she feels familiar, like she knows her but doesn't really know her. Her face is a lot brighter than it was before.

THERAPIST: Do you see her eyes?

YEZDA: Mm-hmm, she's curious and she's very focused at the same time about what's happening. She wants to know who I am and is really drawn to looking at me.

THERAPIST: And when she sees you what does she see? [View of self at the forefront, the therapist uses this opportunity to explicitly inquire about current view of self.]

YEZDA: She sees someone who's really relaxed. She almost has this presence, this energy about her that's really magnetic and she seems happy. Yeah, a little more easygoing and approachable.

THERAPIST: Yeah, that's so beautiful, Yezda, and are there words? Is there any exchange of words?

YEZDA: No, she's just studying me. She's saying, "I want to be that person; I'm watching her so I can learn from her." [Therapist hears a perception of self as a person to be admired, modeled.]

THERAPIST: That's so beautiful, Yezda, and what does your presence say to her? [Therapist follows the client at this level of an engaged encounter, without words.]

YEZDA: My presence says that she can come over, she can be close, she can be with me and that she is me. [Integration and consolidation.]

THERAPIST: That's so beautiful. "You can be with me, and you can be me." You could say that to her, Yezda, you could say that.

YEZDA: "You can be with me, and you can be me, this is attainable, you have it in you, you know how to do the hard work, and you can be happy."

THERAPIST: "And we can be happy together!"

YEZDA: "We can be happy together and we can remember but we don't have to let it hold us back."

THERAPIST: Nice, Yezda, that's beautiful. We can remember but it doesn't actually have to be us, define us, not specific aspects of it, right? The other aspects you're embracing, as a part of you and your definition of you, you're shaping that now. [As the impacts of trauma are disentangled from her story, Yezda can begin to integrate and embrace aspects of her experience that she had disavowed and that had been disavowed, and similarly, begin to shape her future from a more grounded and whole position.]

YEZDA: Yes, and I think those experiences, if anything, have made me more resilient, too. It reminds me of things that Sam has said to me about why he was drawn to me and why he feels close to me. It's because I've had those experiences and that I have a deeper understanding of what it means. He said I know what suffering is, which I've always felt like that may not be the best way of what he was trying to articulate. What I think he meant to say was that I understand and I have overcome, outside of the normal challenging circumstances, and didn't have a network to support me through it like he did. So that's why he felt like we had a common understanding of how to be resilient through hardships.

THERAPIST: It's true, isn't it, Yezda? It's lovely, in many ways, at many times, he says to you, "I see you."

YEZDA: Yeah, he does, when he can clear the space to be present, then he can. (*Smiling.*)

THERAPIST: Yezda, what would he say? What would he see through his eyes when he sees you now? What might he say? [Again, checking in with the perceptions of key others as a means of gauging progress and consolidating gains.]

YEZDA: I think he would say . . . I'm trying to find the right word, he's very influenced, he's . . .

THERAPIST: Inspired?

YEZDA: Yes, and I think it motivates him, too. I think it makes him feel like it's okay to look at these things, and it does inspire him to do the work. I used to always hear from him, "I've already done this work, it's really good if you do it but I've already done it," and now I think he's further from that. I think he acknowledges, now, that it's not a one-time fix. There are new relationships and new circumstances that pull you back to how you were before, and you have to work through that and move forward. So, I think he's more there now, after having seen me go through all this work in the last few years.

THERAPIST: Yezda, that is so beautiful! And you know, Yezda, the other place I go with this is that you've shared your work with so many people around the globe, and it is an inspiration! You are an inspiration, and that little girl is right to look up to you and want to be with you, so nice, that's amazing!

YEZDA: Yeah, I was glad. That's such a special opportunity to do that and to share that with others. There was a part of me that felt like others could benefit from me sharing.

THERAPIST: They do, they are, we are, and we grow with you and beside you, and are honored to be with you as well, Yezda. It's really amazing. And other therapists, of course, around the globe, can be inspired and instructed by you and your beautiful work and your clarity and your strength, all the things that Sam knew.

YEZDA: It's really special to have someone see that side of you, when he sees me and nothing else. I defer back to those experiences we've had in the last few years, since we got engaged and married, when Sam is seeing me and nothing else. It's almost overwhelming to be in that space, but it's nice to have because I've felt like I deserved less than the relationship I have with him. I wouldn't have had that experience with a different partner, which I feel really grateful for.

THERAPIST: Yezda, that's so great! And the more that you take that in, the more that you get to grow one another, which is the goal. You're amazing, Yezda! Are you basking in all of this?

YEZDA: Thank you. It usually takes me about an hour to unpack it but yeah, I am. The relationship with my mom is still unsettling sometimes, but I do feel like I'm progressing with my dad, which is a big reason why I feel more grounded, too, because of that relationship evolving. Just having the space to reflect has been really important to me because I've been so go go go for the last three years and not letting myself think about it. I'd forgotten to really see how far I've come since starting all this. It's been nice, this renewed confidence. I always felt like I was sort of a confident person, since I feel like you have to be when you start a business. I feel like I have a better understanding of what that confidence means for me now, instead of trying to put on a face and act a certain way. I feel it deeply now.

THERAPIST: Yes, you feel it in your feet. I love that you said that Yezda! So great!

In this and other Stage 3 sessions, progress is consolidated. The grips of Yezda's past are now loosened and she is beginning to see her parents in a different light. She is renegotiating her relationship with them, and with her siblings. Memories of her father and his gentle touch, and the many ways he protected her are at the forefront. A new understanding of her mother, and the many ways that her life was restricted by marriage, gender, and discrimination, is evoking a greater sense of compassion, albeit ongoing caution and skepticism in her ability to trust and be close to her mother.

This final stage is marked by increased curiosity in her parents and their respective experiences growing up "worlds away" from each other and from her own world. Her ability to care for herself is noted by those closest to her, especially her husband, as he adjusts to her more direct expression of her needs and her unwillingness to waver from having them met.

Her sense of self now expanded, and her identity more firmly established, Yezda proudly concludes in a Stage 3 session that she has observed herself to be more spontaneous and less serious than she has ever been. As we move through this final stage of therapy, it is with confidence that Yezda will continue to grow and that she will undoubtedly craft the personal and family life she dreamt of as a little girl, but now in a manner that allows her to integrate and hold, not only the difficult aspects of her past, but also her rich cultural history and the fond memories that were once buried.

And, indeed, this is what has happened. In a recent follow-up session, now some years later, Yezda revealed her resolve to create a family tradition of reading *The Night Before Christmas* annually. Now early December, she was preparing to celebrate the first Christmas with her young son, named with homage to her father's cultural background. Her initial attempt to purchase the book was met with nausea as she entered the local bookstore. A deep breath and a few days later she had a shiny copy of the book. On December 24, stockings hung, and the tree decorated, she sat her son on her knee, her phone poised to record the two of them. Her voice cracked initially but she did it, and enjoyed it, then later shared it with her husband. In future years, he can join, too, but for this first time, this was to be done on her terms—a poignant image of agency restored, the reclamation of aspects of childhood lost, and the halting of the intergenerational transmission of trauma.

PLAY AND PRACTICE

For You Personally

Reflecting on the landscape of your life, and the key characters that live in your heart and mind, is there someone that stands out for you as particularly impactful (positive or negative)? Has reading this book shifted your perspective surrounding any of these relationships in any regard? Are there any relationships that you would like to revisit and/or renegotiate? What might this look like? Or, perhaps, are there relationships or anniversaries of key interpersonal events (e.g., loss) that you might like to honor or celebrate? How might that look?

For You Professionally

Whether you are new to EFT and a more attachment-based experiential way of working, or whether this model is familiar to you, we hope that this book has offered something new for you and your practice. Now at the final stage of therapy and as we approach the final chapter, we invite you to journal your experience of this book, your understanding of trauma and how it has transformed using an experiential emotionally focused method. What is new about this model? What seems familiar? How might you adopt this model or integrate aspects of it into your preferred way of working?

KEY TAKEAWAYS

Consolidation of a Secure Base: Key Elements and Sample Questions to Consider

Therapeutic gains are highlighted, consolidated, integrated, and celebrated.
As you look back on the landscape of our work together, what stands out for you?

Shifts in the client's narrative are highlighted.
You said you told this story many times. If you were to tell your story now, what might you say?

New solutions to old problems are identified.
At the beginning of our work together, you spoke about feeling lost. What might you say now?

Shifts in view of self are explored, consolidated, and integrated.
As you stay still with you and look for you, what do you see, where are you? Help me to see what you see.

Shifts in view of and engagement with others are explored, illuminated, and integrated.
If your partner was here, what might they say about what is different and what is the same?

New action tendencies/reactions/behaviors and increased flexibility in response to stress are made vivid and explicit.
At the outset of therapy, you spoke about feeling numb and detached. What might you say now?

Building on the Platform of Felt Security with CARE

Still maintaining attention to the four CARE dimensions:

The client is invited into a vision for the future in terms of goals, aspirations, relationships.

Anniversaries of key events are considered.

Grief is acknowledged and honored.

Key relationships are navigated or renegotiated from a place of security.

Possible symptom aggravation is considered.

9

Addressing Other Types
of Trauma with EFIT

The stories we have shared are among the many we have encountered. We have tried to offer a variety of examples but recognize there
are many more that could be provided. If you have read the preceding
chapters, you have perhaps noticed we have not spoken in any detail of:
first responder trauma; single incident traumas, such as motor vehicle
collisions, natural disasters, and assaults; or traumatic loss. You might
then wonder how the EFIT therapist deals with these types of traumatic
experiences? In short, many of the same principles apply, with some
additional attention to special considerations in each of these areas. We
turn now to a brief snapshot of each of these types of traumas as viewed
through the lens of attachment and addressed with EFIT. Concluding
comments and reflections follow.

FIRST RESPONDER TRAUMA

Here, as with other types of traumas, a safe haven alliance is prioritized,
along with a focus on tuning in and planning treatment with attention to the four dimensions captured by CARE (i.e., Context, Attachment, Relationship, specifically therapeutic alliance, Emotion). Pacing is
guided at the outset and throughout the therapy process by these same
four dimensions, by strengths and resources, by risk factors such as the
likelihood of ongoing exposure to trauma, commonly the case among
first responders, as well as other possible concurrent factors such as
physical injury and rehabilitative efforts or related functioning, and by
family factors such as marital strain, family loss or illness, or parenting

stress. In anticipating the adverse effect of trauma exposure, preexisting vulnerability factors, such as prior loss or trauma, will tend to heighten the risk of negative impact. On the positive side, secure attachment may be a more protective influence. Factors such as these guide interventions and decisions aimed at establishing safety and stabilization in initial sessions. A course of couple therapy may be helpful to bolster the relationship as a resource if there is readiness and willingness on behalf of both partners. Or, if substance misuse has been the main avenue for coping and is likely to be a barrier to the EFIT process, other interventions and/ or adjunct treatment methods might be recommended.

Further, with respect to the four CARE dimensions, specifically "Context" as applied to first responders, or others likely to be exposed to cumulative trauma in the work environment, organizational and leadership factors are highly relevant. For example, if the work culture, and especially leadership, prescribes a "tough it out" and "toughen up" response to heightened stress and trauma exposure, it is less likely that individuals will seek support. If coworkers subscribe to the same philosophy, the collective stigma will probably further limit the likelihood of the responder seeking therapy. If the responder instead turns to alcohol or drugs to numb emotions, support at home is also at risk of being jeopardized. On the other hand, if the work culture and leadership is characterized by high support, open communication about trauma and the potential impacts of cumulative exposure, and the encouragement and provision of opportunity to process the emotional correlates of trauma, buffering effects become more probable. If partners are included in such educational pursuits and similarly offered support, *protective factors are more likely to be cumulative.*

For some clients, cumulative work-related trauma exposure is among the many stressors likely to be ongoing and place mounting demands on personal and relational resources. Manjit poignantly spoke to this in an initial session. As an immigrant to Canada, he had suffered racism and discrimination for years, starting on the school playground. When he put on the police uniform, this only got worse, "Now [he] really was a target." He went on to explain that working in rural Canada only added to the day-to-day stress, making it difficult to separate work from home, and hard for his children to feel any sense of belonging in a predominantly white community, and especially because their "dad is a cop." Organizational and collegial support was limited, and extended family support nil. His brothers and their families had migrated to cities, offering more opportunity for work and community, including religion and culture. The lack of perceived collegial support extended beyond the lack of belonging he felt on the school playground as a child. In a profession relying upon coworkers to serve and protect not only community, but also each other, Manjit felt unsafe. He did not believe that he could rely on his peers.

These and other contextual factors, such as ongoing work-related trauma exposure, were considered in each session and through the therapy process, recognizing that window of capacity is likely to shrink and expand in the context of individuals' daily realities within and outside work.

Manjit worked through key work-related traumatic incidents in the same manner described and illustrated in earlier chapters. Specifically, as the therapist joined with Manjit in revisiting key pivotal work-related incidents and associated scenes, the felt experience was evoked, and the lights were dimmed on the traumatic aspects of the scenario (to avoid retraumatization). Rather, once again, safety and support were illuminated. As Manjit was encouraged to feel what he would have had no space or opportunity to feel at the time of the incident(s), when all his resources were directed to the care and protection of others, encounters were choreographed with various key others, expanding his window of capacity, and his connection with self. With increased capacity and ability to tune into his inner emotional world, he became more able to reach to his wife, and they together worked to build community in rural Canada, and prioritized trips to visit and spend time with family. Manjit provides for us a lovely illustration of the power of increased capacity in leveraging attachment to further expand and grow, and to further increase capacity/window of tolerance and, by extension, resilience.

As described earlier, attachment as represented by CARE also is relevant in guiding and structuring the process, within and between sessions, and over the course of therapy. For example, for the first responder with a secure attachment history, ample self and social resources at work and home, and with a key work-related traumatic incident that is now waking her at night and haunting her by day, perhaps only a few sessions will be required to move with and through the emotion she would have been unable to feel when she was attending to the medical emergency and those directly impacted. On the other hand, for the first responder with a history of childhood trauma and 20 years of service, coupled with reliance on years of emotional numbing and detachment to manage, and now social isolation following divorce, therapy is likely to be longer and to be paced and structured differently. For instance, adjustment to the loss might be at the forefront and the clinical priority at therapy outset. In any case, as alluded to above, the likelihood of continued trauma exposure is a key consideration, along with the benefits of ongoing access to support.

Highly relevant as well are the cumulative impacts of trauma. As in the case of complex or developmental trauma, themes of helplessness, inadequacy, and failure commonly abound among first responders and are often especially pronounced in the case of cumulative exposure to trauma when support is limited and when coping through distancing, numbing, or reactive intensification of emotion has become automatic and reflexive. Consistent with earlier commentary, every incident need not be addressed to begin to reduce symptoms and ultimately restructure self and system. Rather, it can be anticipated that as themes of loss, betrayal, helplessness, at times, futility, are addressed, trauma can be transformed and agency restored.

Caden presented for an initial session some months after a call involving a single motor vehicle accident. A mother and her two sons were driving home from a hockey tournament. Road conditions were poor, and visibility limited. One of the boys, a young teen, was trapped in the vehicle, and the other unconscious when Caden arrived, first on scene. Their mother was distraught and screaming for Caden to do something. It was a rural assignment. Help was on the way, but Caden knew it would take some time. He followed protocol and was ultimately able to release the trapped teen with the help of fire personnel. Paramedics then had both youths and their mother airlifted to the closest major medical facility. A lengthy investigation regarding the mechanics of the accident then followed, with little information forthcoming about the well-being of the family. Some weeks later he was informed both boys had survived and returned to hockey, and their mother similarly recovered from more minor physical injuries. This, along with a departmental debriefing should have been enough, he originally thought, but trauma-related symptoms had persisted over the past months.

Slightly shaking as he recounted events and acknowledged he had not received any counseling despite over two decades of service, Caden pronounced that he had always managed. Most calls had not bothered him but for some reason "this one had really grabbed [him] and stuck with [him]." And now, other calls, involving children and babies, calls he had not thought about for years, had shifted from the recesses to the forefront of his mind. Given indications of a solid and secure personal and relationship history, as well as strong and stable social and organizational support, relatively early in the therapeutic process Caden was able to begin to slow down and revisit key aspects of the scene and feel what he had no opportunity to feel at the time of the traumatic event. He was aware of the parallels between this family and his own, but what he had not realized earlier was his initial encounter with the boys' mother; the look in her eyes and the anguish of her voice was a poignant reminder of the vulnerability of his wife, and that of his own children. In our work with trauma, we often talk about memories triggering emotion but, of course, emotion also carries and cues memory.

Caden now understood the nightmares and intrusive images that were haunting him, and the sweat that was soaking the bed each night. In a therapy session with his wife, he was able to share the impact of the scene but not the details. "I never realized," he said, tears welling in his eyes, "what really hit me and stuck with me were the parallels with our family, and my fears of losing you, or something awful happening to our children." With that, she wept. Relief and gratitude emerged as she wiped away tears, firmly planted her eyes on his, and quietly and softly said, "Thank you."

Their interaction was a powerful reminder of the many conversations we have had with such couples over the years. First responders commonly convey that they avoid sharing their work with partners. They fear their partners will awaken to the same images and feelings that jolt them out of sleep at night and stalk them by day. In response, their partners frequently reply with some version of, "I don't need you to share details with me, I need you to be with me." Indeed, when individuals can share their emotional experience with a trusted supportive other, the impacts of trauma are diminished and relational bonds deepened. This is the antidote to trauma and to the prevention of its often insidious and perpetuating personal and relational impacts.

On the other hand, when the prototypical response to cumulative exposure to work-related trauma and loss is to hide and retreat, to shut down and shut others out, there is no opportunity for trauma processing and closure. Perception narrows. Self-perceptions risk becoming infused with a variety of negative adjectives. View of others constricts to darkness and vigilance for danger. "What's the point?" Aline exclaimed, tears in her eyes and a tone of frustration in her voice. "I feel like I am running from one overdose call to another; am I really making a difference?" Images had begun to haunt her. "I can't unsee what I've seen," she said. Avoiding any such cues in the community on days off, Aline became increasingly isolated. With little to no contact outside work and family, feelings of futility and despair heightened, along with perceptions of self as ineffectual, and the world as dangerous and chaotic.

Indeed, having heard many such stories over the years, it would appear that the built-in trauma to which many first responders are subjected, as they are witness to fatalities, profound human suffering, and the deaths or exploitation of the innocent or vulnerable, particularly children, faces them with an impossible, unsolvable dilemma. It seers into them a truth that most of us can escape looking at close-up, namely, that random life-and-death dangers lurk in the world that cannot be predicted or fully protected against. The illusion that the world is fair, and that, if people act responsibly and carefully, they will be protected, is shattered. Often, in early service years, and particularly before they are parents themselves, first responders may be more capable of warding off this growing realization. However, when they have children of their own—the protection of whom becomes a central driving force in their own lives—what can tend to emerge (at various levels of awareness) is a helpless and inescapable comprehension that they cannot guarantee the safety of those they love and cherish most in the world.

Echoes and memories of historical calls, that had been more in the background prior, can become reawakened and more intrusive. And in reaction to this consuming fear and sense of helplessness, their hypervigilance can, in turn, become more intensified as they try to compensate (and anticipate contingency after contingency) in a doomed effort to prop up the illusion that they can actually control and ensure the safety that, deep down, they know all too well they cannot. As window of capacity continues to shrink with isolation, agitation and irritability are common outcomes, further alienating those they love, partners who can offer care and support, and children who can provide some solace in a world that has become dark.

Common also among first responders, as well as those in other types of professions such as health care, is the risk of *moral injury or distress*. In contrast with Manjit's experience, Trevor felt a strong sense of comradery with his colleagues on the watch. They worked out at the gym, played basketball on Friday afternoons when not on shift, and often enjoyed a beer together at the local pub following games. A younger group, their initiation into the field had included mental health warnings and their commander was similarly conscious of the risks. Debriefings typically followed difficult calls. One such call involved a "possible electrocution." It was a dark fall night. The air was crisp, as were the leaves that covered the ground. When responders arrived, a young male, 17 years old, was yelling for help. He was inside a hydro plant. Having climbed up, he was now lying on the ground by a transformer. He was screaming. Responders were barred from going in. The power company had ordered that no one enter until the power was turned off. It was unsafe to do so. The responders, including Trevor, thus waited and waited, for a full 40 minutes, until hydro workers, who had been responding urgently elsewhere, finally arrived. Meanwhile, inside the plant, the young man kept screaming. He could barely move. He was trying to crawl but couldn't. As Trevor remembered it, there they were—ambulance crew, two police members, and some bystanders—helplessly looking on, 35 feet away from this teen, unable to assist as he continued to lie there badly burned and in obvious agony. People tried to do what they could. They tried to provide calming words. This did not help. Once the power company finally did come and responders could finally enter, the patient was put on a stretcher.

With the patient quickly airlifted to the nearest major medical center, Trevor tearfully summed it up: "That was it, didn't see that kid again." Trevor did phone the young man's closest family member, though, his uncle, and told him what he knew. A couple days later, he received word that the young man had died.

Looking back, Trevor explained, at the outset of therapy three years later, that the screams of the young man were something that he had not been able to get out of his mind. In his words, "I'll always hear that kid screaming for the rest of my life." Just standing there while "the kid begged and pleaded," he said, left him feeling utterly helpless, useless. He had entered this profession to help, and he stood immobilized. A few months after this electrocution call, his police partner who had been at the scene that night went off on medical leave. He did not return.

In terms of himself at the time, Trevor stayed on duty and just pushed through. He still carries a sense of self-blame, though. He still feels like, somehow or someway, he should have done something. If he had been by himself at the scene, without any other responders present, he feels certain that he would have run in, direct command or not, to try to pull the kid out. In his words, "It's hard to face the fact that I didn't do anything, but I didn't. It's hard to live with myself."

"I lost my soul that day," he said, "everything I was raised to believe, and trained to do, I did not do that day. I never took any time off work. I marched on, as we do, and it wasn't until I was transferred to another community that it all came rushing back. Now I am crippled. I can't work. My marriage is a mess. I feel lost." This was the key event, he conveyed. There were many others over the course of his career, but none that impacted him in the way this did. "I don't know who I am anymore," he continued. "If I can't and don't respond as a first responder, then who am I?"

Following these initial sessions and with an understanding that Trevor had a generally positive developmental history and significant support, even in the face of what he described as a crumbling marriage, the therapist was able to move into the Stage 2 process within about 10 sessions. As the therapist joined Trevor in this poignant scene, and as the details came to life, so too, was Trevor able to move into deeper levels of experience, a place he had not yet visited with respect to this significant work-related event. Illuminating the connection between his now older, wiser self and the only few years younger self that was a first responder at the scene that day, the therapist directed Trevor to dim the lights, sounds, smells on the surrounding details of the scene. Key family members, his wife and his brother, also a first responder, were invited into the background as additional resources. As the therapist helped Trevor to assemble, distill, and feel some of the emotion that he was unable to feel at the time of the event, feelings of guilt and shame again emerged. "I should have done something." Maintaining focus and inviting Trevor to stay still in that experience, the therapist asked the older, wiser, now more resourced self to respond to this younger person in the scene. At that point, the intensity of emotion increased significantly. As Trevor sobbed, his voice barely audible, he replied, "If you did, your children wouldn't have a father." As the therapist listened and waited for Trevor to find some relief, he was asked to repeat this same phrase. He did so. "Say it again," the therapist then directed and following this third repetition, Trevor turned to the therapist, "It wasn't my fault. That kid should have never been in there, and it was good none of us followed." Attending also to the presence of his wife and his brother in that imaginal encounter, the therapist asked what he saw and felt from them. They, too, reinforced that he had made the right decisions. He had no choice.

A significant step in resolving the shame associated with this traumatic incident, Trevor then turned his attention to his wife and their marriage in the session. He also felt guilt about the way he had been treating her and responding to their children—he had been agitated and irritable. Following an engaged encounter with his wife in the session and sincere apology, the therapist processed the encounter, noting his wife had been impacted and he relieved. The session was concluded with a Move 5 summary. Recognizing the need to give more attention to his wife and family, Trevor and his wife pursued a course of couple therapy while he continued in individual therapy. As sessions progressed, he became increasingly less agitated and irritable. He even found joy again in the company of family and the sense of purpose that he had felt in his work returned.

SINGLE INCIDENT TRAUMA

Working with single incident trauma is similarly guided by a thorough attachment-based experiential assessment, by the importance of pacing and structuring the therapeutic process, and by choreographing corrective experiences that move clients with and through the emotion that so naturally accompanies intolerable distress, in the company of safe others. As with other types of traumas, impacts are likely to vary as a function of prior experience and exposure, as well as context. Support is again a key factor in resilience, a sense of belonging, and an experience of being seen and heard. As alluded to at the outset of this text and in writings by other authors (e.g., see Bonanno, 2004; Johnson, 2002), posttraumatic growth is possible when a safe haven relational venue is provided for active processing of the emotions associated with those aspects of the traumatic event most personally relevant to the individual exposed, either directly or indirectly. This might be therapy, the arms of a safe and secure key other or others, or a broader national, even global community.

Developmental considerations also are relevant, both in terms of understanding potential impacts and addressing them. Madeline was referred for individual therapy sessions by her lawyer following a motor vehicle collision, about one year prior. She and her then 3-year-old son were enroute to their weekly swim date at the local recreation facility when they were hit in an intersection by a driver who ran a red light. Their vehicle was hit on the passenger side. Her young son was in the back seat, buckled in his car seat, fortunately in the center of the vehicle. He suffered no physical injury, but Madeline had been diagnosed with and treated for whiplash and mild traumatic brain injury. She also had recently undergone a psychological assessment and was diagnosed with generalized anxiety disorder and major depressive disorder, recurrent. Her first episode of depression developed postpartum, following the birth of her son. The second was the diagnosis after the accident. Otherwise, her health had been good, both physically and emotionally, and her attachment relationships positive, historically and currently.

At therapy outset, Madeline described improvement in pain and in various other symptoms such as headaches, fatigue, and concentration difficulties, though such symptoms continued to linger, and she had not yet returned to work full-time. Most pronounced, however, and debilitating, were symptoms of depression and anxiety, along with worry about her young son. His development seemed to be mostly on-target, but he was exhibiting ongoing issues with sleep and with being a passenger in a motor vehicle. With kindergarten only four months away, she was worried about the daily commutes to his French Immersion program, and she was hoping to be well enough to return to work as a lawyer.

The possibility of play or other developmentally appropriate therapy options were considered for her son, as well as some ideas for Madeline and her partner to implement with him. Given his general discomfort with strangers, especially following the accident, Madeline and her partner opted to see what they could do at home. Following the implementation of various suggestions such as sand play with toy cars and drawing, their son was able to express his anger at the other driver, and the fear and vulnerability he undoubtedly felt, sobbing in the arms of his mom whose safety was also jeopardized at that time. With this, Madeline also was able to express in therapy what she had not been able to feel and express at the time of the accident. At that time, her resources were directed elsewhere: the urgency of the circumstances given the probability of oncoming traffic; her physical reality; and the terror surrounding the well-being of her son.

Once again, in the absence of any opportunity to move with and through the emotion that so naturally accompanies traumatic stress, we can all get stuck. Trauma can block emotion. When the consequence is to then accommodate and carry on, avoidance-based strategies can become habitual, reinforcing isolating patterns of being and relating, and maintaining a host of presenting problems. Often, it is these problems or *symptoms* that are the cue to unresolved trauma and the messengers and motivators for self-care.

Angela presented for therapy following a series of panic attacks. Visits to the emergency room of the local hospital revealed no underlying medical concerns. Rather, the physician suggested that she was suffering from anxiety. Counseling was recommended. In initial sessions, Angela described a family and developmental history characterized by love and affection but was now realizing it had been hard for her to take it in. Her younger sister suffered from an eating disorder, a significant worry for her parents, and a preoccupation for the entire family. Family meals and gatherings were colored by concern for her sister. Endeavoring to stay in the background and not cause any additional worry for her parents, Angela did "all the right things." She was an honors student, active on the student council, and after finishing high school, she excelled at university. Following that, she also excelled in business.

In her mid-twenties, she had started to date and was meeting people online, first texting, then a coffee date or two, and taking it further if there was a fit. She had been on a few dates with a man she later stopped seeing due to "bad vibes." Following that, he stalked her. She caught him lurking in her cul-de-sac. Eventually, she called the police. Upon investigation, they asked her if she wanted to do anything, such as put any restrictions in place. She said no. Some months later, though, she arrived home after a night out and found him in her home. She described it as a harrowing experience, and one she had put behind her. He tried to sexually assault her, but she was able to fight back and ultimately escape when police arrived after a neighbor reported suspicious activity next door. She was advised that charges and related investigations would likely be long and arduous. At that point, her father had been diagnosed with terminal cancer and her mother needed her support. She explained away the bruises on her neck and body and ignored the emotional scars. She did not pursue charges. She took time off work. Family patterns were repeated. Her sister continued to struggle, and she became the key support person for her parents.

Five years later, now happily married and planning a family, panic attacks seemed to come out of the blue. As she looked back on the landscape of her life, she recognized a propensity to put her needs aside and care for others but believed that was valiant, a quality to be admired. She also was proud of her ability to "get past" the assault. She did not believe it had impacted her relationship with her husband. She had talked about it with a few friends. It did not seem to affect her.

"Now, when you think about or talk about the assault, what happens inside of you as you return to that space?" the therapist asked. Angela responded with a feeling of confusion. "How did I get into a situation like that? I know bad things happen. That aspect of it isn't what weighs on me, it is the lack of judgment I had. I saw the signs and I didn't take it seriously." As the session continued, Angela was invited to stay still in the experience and tune into what might emerge from her body. She described feeling emotional, "but I never let myself get in that still place. . . . I try to analyze things more, then I don't have to feel as vulnerable, and I don't have to think about the fear I had or the humiliation." Continuing to find space for herself in the terror, fear, humiliation, she identified a place where she gets stuck, the movie stops playing. It was when she walked into the house, her home, and there was someone there. "I don't go to the next step of the event." As she continued to process and reflect upon the experience, now closer to it, she described anger, a sense of injustice, and a feeling of being alone, no one to really turn to, to count on, and there were "bigger, more important things happening." The tone of anger in her voice quickly shifted as she looked down. Appearing solemn, she quietly reflected a recognition of her tendency to put others first.

THERAPIST: Yes, I hear you. Angela, you're so good at describing all this. You're doing amazing. Are you okay to stay with you?

ANGELA: Yes, that's a weird one. . . . I can talk about it with my friends, and I've told my husband, but it's always in a detached way.

THERAPIST: So, part of what this is about, Angela, is making space for you, but not alone. Of course, I will be here with you, and then maybe there are other resources that you could call upon as well, we could just see.

As Angela replayed the movie from start to finish, as she had done with others, in her words "it was as though she was talking about someone else's experience." Now dimming the lights on the perpetrator and the horror of the assault, the therapist returned to and further illuminated the image of her younger self. Her now older, wiser, more resourced self joined with her, the therapist in the background, and her husband close by (but not too close; Angela had invited his presence as support, not as a witness), the therapist asked what she was drawn to do. "I would hold me, hug me." As she imagined doing so, she sobbed.

When asked whether she took it in (Move 4 of the Tango), she replied yes, and noted again that it is difficult to take in the care of others, but she wants to, she knows she needs to. She felt relieved, somehow liberated. Then invited into an encounter with her husband, she revealed capacity to love and be loved, and resolve to make space for her own needs, desires, and vulnerabilities, as well as those of others. Finally, as the session drew to a conclusion, she commented on the clarity she now had surrounding the incident: It was not her fault; she was not remiss in any way; her anger is legitimate. That justice did not occur does not mean that she was not deserving of it.

Demonstrated above are some of the key principles referenced in earlier chapters. That is, in the face of intolerable stress or trauma there are a finite number of ways for us to manage. In the moment, we either *freeze or flee*, and it is in the aftermath that impacts either fester or fade, depending on our social resources, and on our capacity to reach and be held and to move with and through the emotion that so naturally accompanies traumatic experience.

Our attachment histories often set the tone but are not set in stone. Just as trauma can dramatically shift our views of ourselves and others toward insecurity, and especially when it is chronic or cumulative, so too, can new experiences of comfort and care in times of need move us in the direction of secure attachment. Indeed, as Angela was able to feel in the company of safe others what she was previously unable to feel, what was unsafe to feel, at the time of the traumatic event, this provided a sense of relief, liberation, and naturally led to the challenging of some longstanding relational patterns related to love and being loved. Any self-blame she carried was let go, and the sense of injustice she felt was amplified and legitimized!

Such was the case with Madeline as well. Opportunity to move with and through the emotion she had no opportunity to feel at the time of the accident, and for her young son to do the same, allowed them both to move back into a felt sense of safety and security, with themselves and key others, and in the world more generally. Other types of single incident trauma, such as natural disasters, are commonly shared with family, neighbors, and communities, often ameliorating the impacts given opportunity for shared experience, as well as external support from various sources such as first responders, government agencies, the media, even funding resources from citizens near and far. In such circumstances, the requisite for processing is often met—opportunity to feel and share with safe others the *felt experience* associated with the traumatic stress. An additive protective or resiliency factor might be the experience of being seen and heard in a time of need by a broader social network.

Also often noteworthy in the case of single incident trauma is the absence of shame, and when shame or a close relative such as guilt exists, it is unlikely to pose the same degree of barrier as shame that evolves in the context of chronic exposure to trauma through early childhood years. Specifically, for example, though Madeline might revisit the moments prior to and surrounding the accident with guilt and remorse given the impact on her son, such thoughts are more readily combatted than those associated with a shame-infused definition of self. The key difference being *what I did (or didn't do)* versus *who I am.*

TRAUMATIC LOSS

Grief is an existential reality to be lived through, a process. As George Bonanno and others have demonstrated through a host of empirical studies, most people will find their way through grief to growth and resilience on their own terms, with their own timelines, and their own guidelines (Bonanno, 2019). We also recognize, however, that much like growth, the organic grief process can get thwarted in the same way. That is, when the mobilizing force of emotion is blocked, so too, is grief, and by extension, the capacity to move through the loss and back into growth and resilience. Grief is a process that enlivens self and system, often after a period of stagnation in the wake of loss, and especially traumatic loss. As described earlier, all trauma involves loss. Not all loss involves trauma, but when it does, it can be a barrier to moving with and through the emotion that so naturally accompanies loss.

Before discussing traumatic loss in detail, we first offer some considerations and assumptions central to our understanding of and work with loss.

Guiding Assumptions and Considerations

In joining with clients surrounding loss, we do so again with attention to CARE and with respect to our attachment frame. As described in greater detail below, and again highlighted by Bonanno's work, most people move through their unique grief journeys back into growth and resilience, needing only an attuned companion to accompany them. In other cases, clients might get stuck. Offering some guiding assumptions and considerations, the EFT model again offers a solution.

Loss Is Destabilizing

From an attachment point of view, disorganization, and disorientation in the face of loss is a natural response, consistent with our hard-wired psychobiological system. This system moves us to seek proximity with central attachment figures during times of need. When those others are accessible, responsive, and engaged, our nervous systems are soothed, and we can continue to explore, learn, and grow in this safe haven of connection. When those others are not available, our propensity is to protest and to respond with a host of emotional reactions including anxiety, sadness, anger, and longing for our loved one. In the case of loss to death, these reactions are not just likely, they are expected.

Our key relationships are central to who we are—to our identity. In secure relationships, they are central to an ever-evolving sense of self. It makes sense then, that when we lose someone we love, and especially if that loved one is someone we have relied on extensively, this naturally shakes our foundation, rocks our emotional balance, and leaves us feeling uncertain of our identity and of our place in the world. If loss of a key other is sudden and traumatic, it can be even more destabilizing and disorienting.

This notion of disorganization and disorientation was beautifully depicted in an artist's account of love and loss as revealed in her stained-glass artwork. She indicated that she had been doing stained glass work for years, always of a similar design with consistent features. Specifically, her work was always linear, with carefully selected pieces of glass of different shape, size, and texture, and always with a row somewhere in the piece with colored cubes, selected to represent the colors of the rainbow, always carefully placed in the correct order. Her eyes filled with tears as she explained that it took her months to return to her studio following the loss of her husband. Still months following that first return to this aspect of her life, she was tidying her studio when she noticed that something was amiss, the colors of the rainbow were out of order, much like her life felt at the time, and continued to feel.

Loss Inherently Involves Change

As David Kessler, well-known grief expert, states, all loss has in common change. With change, things can feel out of order. There can be missing pieces. An emptiness—a void.

Even if we have chosen change, such as a decision to break off a relationship, or to move to a new city, with change comes loss, and with loss comes grief. Change can be hard. It is even harder when we have not chosen it.

As described beautifully by Joan Didion (2007) in her book surrounding sudden loss, *The Year of Magical Thinking,* "Life changes in the instant. The ordinary instant. . . . Grief turns out to be a place none of us know until we reach it. We anticipate (we know) that someone close to us could die, but we do not look beyond the few days or weeks that immediately follow such an imagined death. We misconstrue the nature of even those few days or weeks. We might expect if the death is sudden to feel shock. We do not expect this shock to be obliterative, dislocating to both body and mind. We might expect that we will be prostrate, inconsolable, crazy with loss. We do not expect to be literally crazy, cool customers who believe their husband is about to return and need his shoes."

For those of us who have loved and lost, we know this to be so. We naturally and unnaturally expect our loved one to appear, for our coffee to show up on the bedside as it has each morning for the past 20 years, for our pet to be waiting outside the bathroom door when we walk out of it, for the screech of that violin to pierce the quiet of the night once again. We long for what has been lost, for that which matters most, and for that which has provided us comfort in the dark and joy in the light. This is the human condition.

As change agents working with trauma, we can anticipate loss. As highlighted earlier, and illustrated in the chapter featuring Karen and Randy, when people get in touch with what is possible, what is safety and security in the arms of another, so too, does the rush and agony of loss come forward. As these moments of change toward secure connection are illuminated, so too, must the grief associated with lost time, opportunities, relationships be honored. Again, here and in other areas of loss and grief, we meet clients in their current and historical context, with curiosity and respect, attending and attuning to their unique way of grieving in the context of their family, community, or culture, and in the broader sociocultural context.

Grief Has a Natural Rhythm

Many of us have heard our friends, our loved ones, our clients talk about grief coming in waves. Naturally, if we expect our partner to return for their shoes, our attachment system is going to be primed for proximity seeking. Longing is likely.

Following loss, especially sudden, traumatic, and unexpected loss, we can expect our hard-wired psychobiological system to be fully engaged, but we also can expect the propensity to *look for and long for* our loved one to be punctuated by periods of reprieve—we turn away, rather than toward the pain. This oscillation between proximity seeking and avoidance, this tendency to feel and address grief in waves is what allows us to eventually get back to living again, initially eating and sleeping and later, engaging in other aspects of life.

As the everyday world of activities is recovered, so too, can our attachment hierarchies be reordered or edited, paving the way for other important pillars to share space in higher ranks of the hierarchy while also holding onto the life we've lived, the story we've told, and the relationships we've nurtured, including that with the deceased.

As the physical pain and agony of grief shifts and turns toward a new life as exemplified by the person's ability to somehow reconcile the loss—to accept and make sense of it in a way that is no longer crippling—to go on living again, there is room for our lost loved one and there is increased space for *something* or *someone new*.

Grief Can Be a Frequent Visitor

In our work with couples, we say that in securely attached love relationships, we fall in love over and over again. With love comes the risk of loss, and some version of this same *revisiting* is true with grief. *Following the loss of a loved one, grief becomes an expected and unexpected guest at various times throughout our lives.* We can anticipate that grief might emerge at anniversaries and birthdays, but we also, at times, can be jolted by the sudden grip of grief, get caught off guard, even years after a loss, and even when that loss has been grieved and woven into the tapestry of past and present. Attachment theory and science would tell us to welcome and embrace it as part of our love stories and of our shared humanity.

Edoardo found himself living again. He was laughing at the soccer pitch with his pals of 30 years when a young man about the age that his son would have been suddenly appeared. Also laughing, beer and popcorn in hand, the young man shuffled past and into his seat. Same curly black hair and that same light-hearted air of confidence. Edoardo's heart sank. The color left his face. Time stood still. The punch to his gut left that same familiar feeling of nausea. He dropped his own popcorn to the ground. A cascade of emotions then followed: sorrow; an aching longing; then a moment of anger followed by guilt. "I should not be here. My son should be sitting in this seat," he thought, a thought that had passed through his mind many times before but that had become less frequent and less intense in recent years. The shift in mood was palpable. Moments later, Edoardo was back; his friend's arm now draped around his shoulder, he could feel the warmth of his touch. We know from the series of hand-holding studies we conducted that touch literally soothes the nervous system (Johnson et al., 2013). The color returned to Edoardo's face as he started to breathe again. He quietly whispered, "Joe would have loved this game. He should be here." "Yes. Yes, he should be," his friend answered.

Accompanying Clients through Grief with CARE

Guided by CARE, we recognize that although grief is a part of the human condition—if we love we will grieve—the way we each grieve will be as unique as the individual grieving and that which is being grieved. As we join with our clients, we get to know them and their loved ones, including those they lost. We join with them, experientially, at their dinner tables, at work, and in their spiritual, sports, dance, music, and other communities. We get to know the cast of characters that live in our clients' minds, and we get to know them in the context in which they live and have lived, including the broader sociocultural and inter-generational contexts.

We are curious about the relationship with the deceased, the security of their relationship, the degree to which they moved together and apart, and the extent of their reliance on one another in times of need. We are curious about what the loss means to them, what is lost, and what can be found.

What can be *found,* you might be wondering? From an attachment perspective, when we feel safe and secure in the arms of those we love, we can access them from near and far, when they are away for work or out buying groceries. When they have been a pillar of security and shared in our joy of a job well done, our baby's first steps, or been there for us during a time of need, when our parents died, or when we lost our job, we can call upon a mental representation of these key others. We may not hear their voices, but we can find their words. We know the advice that would be given, the look of compassion, and the warmth of their presence.

Through grief and loss and into growth and resilience yields the possibility of what attachment theorists sometimes describe as a symbolic source of security, commonly referred to as a *continuing bond* in the grief literature. Such terms capture what playwright Robert Anderson wrote more than a decade after the death of his first wife about her continued place in his life: "I have a new life. . . . Death ends a life, but it does not end a relationship, which struggles on in the survivor's mind toward some final resolution, some clear meaning, which it perhaps never finds" (1974, p. 77). This final clause in the sentence also seems to represent and legitimize the experience of mourners. Grief has no timeline. Love lasts a lifetime. There is no expiration date on love.

This notion of a continuing bond also was illustrated in the earlier chapter featuring Sierra. As we joined Sierra in her grandmother's garden, the security of their bond, and the power of her grandma in offering support was palpable. Indeed, some months later in the therapy process,

Sierra shared the realization that her grandmother symbolically attended her graduation ceremony in celebration of her master's degree, smiling and eyes twinkling as she watched and listened while Sierra spoke at the podium in traditional regalia. Indeed, these continuing bonds can be called upon as resources during times of need and during moments of celebration.

In EFIT, we carefully track this natural biologically driven organic process, as well as the variety of emotions that accompany it. In some circumstances, people come to us looking for a trustworthy other to join them on their own self-initiated, self-prescribed journey of grief. In other cases, people feel stuck. They describe feelings of immobility, paralysis, lack of motivation, depression, anger, anxiety, guilt, shame. The combination, frequency, and intensity of such emotions vary as a function of numerous factors, including, for example, pre- and post-loss factors, such as prior loss or trauma, as well as circumstantial factors such as the type of loss and the nature of the relationship with the deceased, and a host of other variables such as the grieving individual's natural propensity to cope and the breadth and depth of their social network.

These are natural emotions, common responses to loss, so how do people get stuck? Key from an EFIT point of view, as described earlier, we assume that we are hard-wired for connection and that we are intrinsically motivated to grow. Once again, if we consider emotions, the motivating force that moves us when we get stuck, most typically, is because we have not moved through the emotions associated with some key event, perhaps a trauma or loss event, or it could be a relationship event or set of events. Caught in an absorbing state of being triggered, then reflexively and automatically shutting down, lashing out or some combination of both, we remain stagnant. Our world shrinks rather than expands. Growth is foiled rather than fostered.

Identifying Blocks to Mobilize Grief

In working with loss, after joining with and creating a safe haven alliance with our clients and getting to know them and their worlds, we then move to understand the prototypical ways in which they move (or don't move) through the world emotionally and relationally. We help them to identify their own pattern of trigger and response and the blocks or barriers that are preventing them from living fully. As in the case of trauma, we help them assemble, order, and distill their emotional experience, then set up encounters with key others to help them move through the emotions that might have been intolerable or unsafe to feel at the time of these pivotal events, or perhaps there was no space to feel them given that all their resources were focused elsewhere. Such was the case with Jane. She had been there to support her husband Bob when he was diagnosed with terminal cancer, when he decided to go ahead with MAID (Medical Aid in Dying), and even in those final moments together as the physician carried through with his wishes. It was there she was stuck. Her resources diverted elsewhere, toward her life partner and their adult children, she held her breath. At therapy outset she was still not breathing. As therapist and client revisited this scene, Jane was able to find herself and her experience and share her own reality. She did not want to let him go. As she felt his firm hands wrap around her arms, she sobbed. She grieved. She had been there for him, and now he was there for her.

Naturally embedded in an emotional process as it is, grief is not paralyzing. To the contrary, it is mobilizing. Seen through an attachment and EFIT lens, as people move with and through the emotions inherently associated with grief, they find themselves and their inner emotional worlds and are better equipped to seek and find security in others and build a new life while retaining the old. As Jane continued to move forward with her own life, new grandchildren, a puppy, and new hobbies and interests, she shared family news with Bob. She also revealed that she had told him that the cedar box that held his ashes, engraved with an eagle atop, would have a companion box to one day hold her ashes. It, too, would bear the crest of an eagle. Side by side, the eagles would face each other, allowing them to hold one another's gaze. She concluded, "Eagles mate for life."

Addressing Trauma to Make Space for Grief

Circumstances involving traumatic loss are again informed by attachment science and the three-stage EFIT process, and by the overarching goal of restabilization (following a natural period of destabilization in the wake of loss), and a restructuring of self and system to accommodate the loss. For some, working through traumatic impacts and associated symptoms kickstarts the organic grief process, making way for something or someone new, and a restructuring of the individual's attachment hierarchy. For others, and especially those with prior histories of loss and/or trauma with no resolve, careful titration of interventions is guided by person and process, and addressing current loss can help to address losses of the past.

Mary and her husband of over 20 years were referred by their family physician following the loss of their daughter in a tragic motor vehicle accident. They got the knock on the door that all parents fear and dread. Mary has not slept since, while Peter has found refuge in his church community. Mary has never felt the same sense of belonging. This is the community Peter grew up in and right now, she just wants to hide.

They both attended the hospital but viewed their daughter from different angles as she lay in the bed. They visited the wreckage site to retrieve
her personal belongings. As they shared memories, Mary didn't see their
daughter, she saw the blood-filled bag hanging from the bed, and the
motor vehicle seat spotted with blood and covered in their daughter's
beautiful hair. These same images were waking her at night and jolting
her by day, interrupting any possibility of grief.

As Mary was able to revisit these aspects of her experience (carefully choreographed to avoid retraumatization and to offer support as
illustrated with various other clients), and rather than numbing out and
detaching, by sharing memories and images and associated felt experience, trauma was transformed and she was able to begin to grieve her
daughter. As grief was mobilized, she turned to her husband in new
ways. On one sunny morning she accompanied him to church. "Life will
never be the same," she said. "I will never attend her wedding or hold
her children, but I can now hold fond memories of our time together."
The horror of the tragic accident no longer at the forefront, Mary was
able to find and share the many ways her daughter blessed their family
and community. And now, she conveyed, she could get back to living, to
caring for her other children and now grandchildren.

In other cases, unresolved relationship trauma might be a barrier to
grief. Again, our AIRM protocol informs us and attention to the four
CARE dimensions guides the process. Timothy's divorce from Samantha
10 years prior had been fraught with legal bills and conflict surrounding
the division of assets, custody, and access to their young children. Now
in the wake of Samantha's sudden death to heart failure, their two teenage children were struggling. Still angry, it was hard for Timothy to be
there for his children, and hard for him to get close to any feelings of
grief and loss. He did not want to revisit this all over again. In his mind,
he had erased the 20 years of his life they had been together. He had
"moved on." Now he was faced with dealing with her again. Resentment
was at the forefront.

As the therapist worked with Timothy to disentangle and order the
array of emotions he was feeling, he was able to move past the resentment to the anguish he never allowed himself to feel when Samantha had
the affair that spelled the end of their marriage. He also recognized that
he had been remiss in their relationship, focusing on work and providing for the family in material ways, at the neglect of his wife's emotional
needs. In an in-session imaginal encounter with his ex-wife, he was now
able to see and feel the pain she had unsuccessfully tried to share in earlier years. He apologized for his neglect of key aspects of their marriage
and, she, in turn, apologized for betraying him and the impact on their
family. Liberated to some degree from this loss, Timothy was able to

make more space for the current circumstances. As his children shared fond memories and photos, he too was able to revisit earlier times without anger and resentment, but instead with pride in the foundation that they as a couple had together provided for their young children.

CONCLUDING COMMENTS AND REFLECTIONS

Once again, in all types of traumas, attachment science offers a map and EFT provides a method. Safety and stability are the clinical priorities at therapy outset, and interventions are aimed at helping individuals to feel what might have previously been unacceptable, intolerable, or somehow inappropriate to feel at the time. The EFT Tango is used to propel clients through the three-stage process. Change occurs through corrective emotional experiences or identity epiphanies, leading to deep and sustainable change and a platform for ongoing growth and resilience. These changes are highlighted, consolidated, and integrated in session over the course of treatment and in the final stage of therapy.

In all cases, we would assert that attachment is at the core of our understanding of the impacts of trauma, and it is at the level of attachment that deep and sustainable change occurs, affording the individual a return to growth, or perhaps in the case of longstanding early developmental trauma, kickstarting the organic growth process in deep ways for the first time. We would also argue that without change at this level, second order change as described earlier, vulnerability is not only probable (as it is in the case of a prior trauma history coupled with clinically relevant symptoms), but also inevitable. Second order change, that associated with restructuring of self and system, provides hope and resilience.

PLAY AND PRACTICE

For You Personally

None of us escapes loss. When you have loved and lost, who did you turn to? Who was your companion in the grief process? Of course, it might not have been a therapist. It might have been a friend, a family member, a spiritual figure, or some other attachment figure. Is there a loved one you carry with you, a continuing bond, a source of solace during times of stress, and a cheerleader in key moments of success? Would it be helpful to further illuminate this individual in your life (as Sierra did her grandmother in an earlier chapter)? If yes, how might you do so?

For You Professionally

We have now reached the end of this aspect of our journey together, the last chapter in this book. How will you apply what you have learned to your work? How has it changed your work or further solidified your current way of working? Identify and write down three key takeaways that you may use in your work?

KEY TAKEAWAYS

Special Considerations in Working with First Responder Trauma

Anticipate ongoing exposure to trauma and variable capacity.
Attend to the possible impacts of cumulative exposure to trauma.
Consider moral distress or injury.
Anticipate symptom resurgences given probable trauma exposure and heightened vulnerability.

Special Considerations in Working with Single Incident Trauma

Consider developmental, risk, and protective factors in case conceptualization and in structuring the process.
Shame is unlikely to present the same level of barrier observed in the context of developmental trauma.

Guiding Assumptions and Considerations in Working with Loss

Loss is destabilizing.
The nature and security of the relationship matters.
Change inevitably accompanies loss.
All trauma involves loss.
Grief has a natural rhythm.
The organic grief process is characterized by oscillation between proximity seeking and avoidance.
Grief can be a frequent visitor, an expected and unexpected guest.
Clients are accompanied through grief with CARE.
Many clients only require a companion in grief, a trusted and trustworthy other. Some require help with unblocking the natural grief process.
In traumatic loss, trauma is addressed to make space for grief.
The AIRM protocol informs resolution of relationship trauma to make way for grief.

Appendix

Moving through the
Three Stages of EFIT

Herein is a quick summary of the therapy process for your future reference. First, we provide an overview and then we introduce a client, Marjorie. From there we outline the three-stage process with reference to Marjorie, as well as to other clients you have met earlier in this book, as applicable.

THREE STAGES OF EFIT:
WHAT ARE THE ANTICIPATED OUTCOMES?

As a temporary attachment figure, an instrument in the process, we use ourselves, our personhood, and our voices to attune to our clients in creating a safe haven alliance. We track, reflect, validate. In Stage 1 of the treatment, as we put up a mirror for our clients, they begin to see themselves. And, just as importantly, they feel seen. They begin to better understand trigger and response, their prototypical way for moving in the world emotionally and relationally, and how these patterns keep them stuck.

We then help our clients move into frightening, alien, and unacceptable emotion. As the frightening becomes manageable, the alien familiar, and the unacceptable tolerable, so too, do prototypical strategies become less restrictive. The space between trigger and response widens. Reactivity moves toward flexibility. Windows of tolerance expand. Narratives become more coherent. Emotional balance improves.

As we move into Stage 2 of the process, with this increased capacity clients move more deeply into core vulnerabilities and stay longer, allowing felt shifts in their experience to occur in relationship, followed by new meaning making and new perceptions. Using the Tango as a guide in this bottom-up process, Moves 1 and 2 involve organizing and structuring the session, and assembling, distilling, and deepening emotion. Move 3 offers opportunity to harness the power of relationship to choreograph corrective emotional experiences or identity epiphanies and Moves 4 and 5 afford opportunity to process and integrate, and consolidate these changes. As change occurs at these deep levels, trauma is transformed. Clients find their agency.

The protective strategies that have become their prisons are unlocked. As the organic growth process is unblocked, clients can continue to move into a felt sense of security with themselves and others. The process of healing through EFT is now in full motion with clear and tangible signs of growth within and between sessions. In this Stage 3 process, the therapist guides the client in owning and knowing the gains that have been made and how best to build on them.

INTRODUCTION TO MARJORIE

Marjorie sat across from the therapist, her arms folded and her forehead creased. She appeared frustrated only minutes into the session. "Nice to meet you Marjorie," the therapist said in a soft slow voice, her own body language intentionally inviting, but not too close or intrusive (sitting back, arms resting on the arms of her chair, giving Marjorie lots of space). "Did you have any thoughts or expectations about what this initial meeting might be like?" Marjorie looked down. "Do you know what you are hoping you might gain from our time together?" the therapist said, titrating her voice and distance to create safety. Marjorie glanced out of the corner of her eye with a look of mistrust. "I don't know," she retorted. She had been referred by her lawyer and had no experience in therapy.

The therapist sat silent for a moment, then said, with a look of empathy, engaged, fully present and curious, "It's okay, you can take your time. You can let me know if there are ways that I can make this more comfortable for you." With this, Marjorie softened. Her forehead relaxed and she looked slightly tearful. The therapist's eyes also swelled with tears. They both sat silently for a moment, looking at each other, both likely wondering what might come next.

As this initial session progressed, Marjorie began to exhibit greater ease. Now in her 50s, she acknowledged that she had been struggling for years and that nothing had helped. She had never been to therapy, but she had pursued various types of medically and other-based interventions. She did not feel particularly hopeful.

As she shared her story, she conveyed a developmental history of trauma and loss beginning in early adolescence. Prior to that, in her words, "life was bliss," until her mother died suddenly in a motor vehicle collision when Marjorie was 13 years old. Marjorie and her brother had been in the vehicle but escaped unharmed. Their mother died on impact. There had been a service, lots of community support initially, then nothing. Following that, Marjorie's father retreated into his work and a stiff drink or two nightly. Her younger brother similarly escaped, much of his time engrossed in sports or video games. Marjorie, too, retreated into a world of books and art. A self-proclaimed introvert, she had a few select friends but tended mainly to rely on intimate relationships, some with teenage girls, some boys, some positive, some not. Particularly noteworthy in her story was an account of a young man who had systematically exploited her sexually, verbally, and emotionally. This relationship lasted about two years, between 16 and 18 years of age. As soon as she graduated from high school, she left home to pursue a career in art. She met and married a beautiful woman in her mid-20s. Initial years were wonderful, but their relationship ended after 10 years when her partner had an affair due, her partner claimed, to Marjorie's inaccessibility and propensity to withdraw.

Now in a relationship with a man for the past 13 years, she is a stepmother to two teenage children (his children from a previous marriage). Marjorie described him as kind and supportive. "He says he loves me, but I don't believe him." She worries she will lose him, that he will give up trying, and that he will give up on her, them. She is angry and irritable, chronically agitated. Intimacy has waned since Marjorie was in a motor vehicle accident about four years ago. She has since been diagnosed with posttraumatic stress disorder, major depressive disorder, and fibromyalgia. In her words, her career has tanked. She has not been able to paint for four years. She wants help.

STAGE 1: STABILIZATION

In Stage 1 of EFIT, the therapist actively creates a safe haven alliance. As the therapist joins with the client in understanding the client's story/narrative and tunes in and finds focus, so too, does the client begin to make sense of current experience in context, specifically, symptoms and relational challenges. Protective strategies are understood as adaptive in specific contexts but potentially blocks (to self and other) in the current context. Tracking, reflection, and validation is the EFIT therapist's version of psychoeducation. For example, "It makes sense, Marjorie, that you would retreat when you lost your mom. It sounds like that was the only thing you could do. There was no one there, for their own reasons likely, that we might not ever fully understand. Your dad and brother retreated into their work and activities. It was hard for your dad to keep the family together. But now, what I hear you saying is your partner wants to be close, wants to be there for you, but it is hard for you to take that in, to trust it, to believe in it."

As the therapist gently nudges the client toward felt experience, the aim of doing so is made explicit. Transparency provides agency. Agency is always important, but especially for those who have not had it in earlier times in their lives. For clients who tend to reactively intensify emotion, it can be helpful to slow the process to bring clients closer to themselves and their experience (e.g., shifting voice tone, body language). For those who tend to rely on numbing or shutting down, inviting clients to be still with themselves and their experience might be useful. Once again, as aptly highlighted by Bessel van der Kolk, in *The Body Keeps the Score* and which might be the gateway to emotion, to felt experience. For example, "Marjorie, as you tune into that time in your life, and I will be there, too, what do you remember about your mom? Can you find her? Do you see her? What happens inside of you as you begin to get closer to that time in your life?" If this is difficult to access, as is often the case, the therapist might invite Marjorie to focus on any bodily sensations. "As you stay still with yourself, and I'm here, too, do you notice anything in your body, a tightness, a knot, anything at all?" Some clients will need such hints surrounding bodily sensation, while others will not, and some will be able to access and name their emotional experience.

Notice also here that the therapist explicitly names the presence of a safe other. If there are other safe others to bring forward, the therapist also draws attention to that key other (e.g., could be a deceased grandparent, a spiritual figure). In other cases, a resource, such as a love of art or music, might be called upon at various points in the therapy process, or the therapist might inquire about moments of confidence and competence (e.g., in sports). Most often, and especially when the view in the rearview mirror of a client's life is mainly dark and grim, such moments will have receded into the background. Persistent inquiry and curiosity can bring strengths and resources closer to the forefront. Corrective emotional experiences that broaden and deepen capacity through the Stage 1 and into the Stage 2 process will also allow for easier access to and acknowledgment of strengths and resources.

In some cases that involve significant and longstanding exposure to trauma, especially that occurring early in childhood and persisting through development, the therapist might stay in Tango Move 1 for a significant period, helping the client to create a coherent narrative and increased awareness of the origins of and logic surrounding prototypical strategies for being and relating (distancing from self and others). In other cases, clients might have a generally coherent narrative and an understanding of what triggers them (e.g., feeling dismissed) and their likely response (e.g., lashing out or shutting down). Very often, however, clients have not had the opportunity to slow this sequence down and identify the elements between trigger and response (i.e., perception, meaning, and bodily response). It is here that the therapist might then focus and help the client assemble/order emotion, creating both increased awareness and coherence. In the case of Marjorie, for example, any threat of abandonment or loss might evoke withdrawal, shutting down, and a feeling of being alone (meaning making) and unable to trust others (immediate perception/threat). As she focuses on her body, she might find a tightness in her throat, that she is holding her breath (bodily sensation), "waiting for the shoe to drop." As the therapist stays still with her in this experience, inviting her to breathe while the therapist breathes, too, feelings of sadness and grief quietly emerge. Marjorie becomes tearful and lowers her head.

Once clients have gained awareness and coherence or once the therapist has assessed such existing capacity, and resources are identified and brought to the forefront, the therapist might consider choreographing engaged encounters (Move 3 of the Tango) with the aim of challenging prototypical strategies, and/or assessing access/proximity to self. For example, "Good Marjorie, I hear you, that's good. What I hear you saying is when you move into your family home, your bedroom, picturing that time in your life, things look blurry. But as you stay still, there is a bit more visibility, like the flowy flowered curtains, and as you stay still with you, do you see you? Are you there?" This initial venture into felt experience might then be revisited, the scene now clear and the ultimate beacon in sight: a felt sense of security with self and others typified by the capacity to tune into internal experience; the ability to share that experience and related needs, fears, longings, and vulnerabilities coherently and directly with others; and the capacity to give and receive love.

In this scenario, if Marjorie were to be able to find herself, the therapist might invite older, wiser, adult Marjorie to look into the young adolescent's eyes, and might ask, "What are you drawn to do/say?" Alternatively, another attachment figure might be chosen. Notice, at times, the therapist follows and at other times, the therapist leads. Marjorie might then say, "Just be with her, sit beside her." Again, centered on the goal of EFIT, the therapist might ask, "Can she feel you? Does she take in your care and support?" (Move 4 of the Tango). If the answer is yes, then the therapist integrates, consolidates, and celebrates this gain with a Move 5 of the Tango. For example, "Do you see what just happened, Marjorie? Do you see what you just did? When you took the risk of going back to that difficult time in your family home, and stayed still in your experience, in your body, rather than reflexively moving away from it, shutting down and retreating, the thing that happened is that you found some of those feelings you were unable to feel during that difficult time. You found you, and when I asked you what you were drawn to do, you automatically and reflexively moved toward that younger you, something she didn't have at that time, again for lots of good reasons. Your dad and brother also were in their own corners of the house. You said that she could feel you there, but she wouldn't look at you. That's okay, Marjorie, that's how this works. The more that you/she can feel what would have been unsafe, intolerable, too overwhelming to feel at the time of that tragic accident and loss, but not feel it alone—none of us encounter vulnerability alone—the more that you can find you, and the more she/you can begin to trust that maybe others can be there for you during a time of need."

As therapist and client revisit pivotal moments likely to have been instrumental in shaping view of self and other, and establishing and maintaining affect regulation strategies (and thereby impacting capacity/flexibility), prototypical strategies are challenged, along with existing views of self and other. Recognizing that key events can often be organized and understood around attachment-based themes (e.g., fear of abandonment, feeling alone, being betrayed), it is not necessary to recall every impactful event, nor is it necessary to revisit each event. Just as traumatic experience can have a ripple effect on attachment security, so too, can corrective emotional experiences begin to dissolve blocks and protective strategies and create increased flexibility in views of self and system (other). As this occurs within session, change also occurs between sessions and can be monitored. For example, in the case of Marjorie, we would anticipate shifts in capacity to tune into her internal experience and share it with a key other, such as her husband. The therapist might explicitly gauge such progress through engaged encounters in session or through inquiry. In some cases, as described earlier in this book, a course of couple therapy might be considered as a means of supporting the individual therapy process.

To summarize, by the end of Stage 1, the following can be anticipated:

- increased awareness of patterns of strategies for managing stress and of interactions with key others;
- a more coherent narrative increasingly linked to symptoms and to the way client defines self and others;

- improved emotional balance/wider window of tolerance (more flexibility, less numbing/reactivity, greater capacity to move into and through emotion);
- a reduction in symptoms (e.g., less anxiety, depression, intrusive symptoms such as flashbacks, nightmares, irritability, and anger);
- increased awareness of fears, longings, vulnerabilities, and their legitimacy;
- improved exploration (ARE: Accessibility/Openness, Responsiveness, and Engagement) with self and key others, more discovery-oriented;
- movement toward more self- and other-acceptance and compassion;
- increased access to key elements of models of self and other and improved flexibility; and
- a new sense of hope and self-efficacy.

STAGE 2: RESTRUCTURING SELF AND SYSTEM

Against this backdrop of increased flexibility and openness, the EFIT therapist can pitch interventions at deeper levels with the understanding that clients have increased capacity to move more readily and deeply into felt experience and remain present for longer periods, creating opportunity for restructuring of self and system through corrective emotional experiences or identity epiphanies. In this state of flow, for example, the client might feel viscerally and experientially for the first time. We can see this in the work with Sierra.

"It's not my fault," Sierra said. "I now realize that though I was the common denominator in all those dramas that shaped my life, it wasn't because I was bad. And I also now realize that my mom did her best—she was a single mom and my dad had his own difficult experiences growing up." Here the therapist might reflect to consolidate such gains: "You can begin to see and understand yourself and others in new ways, with more compassion and understanding. That's right Sierra, it was not your fault, it could never be the fault of a tiny child. There is nothing you could have done to deserve the neglect, poverty, and deprivation you described in our early meetings together. And I recognize that you also are beginning to see and understand the key people in your life differently, as well as some of the ways their experiences impacted them."

At times, these shifts in view of self are subtle and incremental, and at other times, they appear as watershed moments in the therapy process. Whatever the case, the therapist follows and leads, unblocking barriers to growth and connection, and highlighting and illuminating new experiences of self as confident and competent. As therapy progresses and capacity deepens and broadens, at times, new memories emerge. Again, the therapist follows and leads with curiosity not assumption, with the overarching goal of bringing clients home to themselves and their experience. In some cases, these new memories may simply complete an incomplete picture of the client's narrative, and at other times, they might represent a previously inaccessible aspect of experience that was deeply intolerable but defining. In this latter case, the therapist would join the client in revisiting this experience, feeling what was intolerable to feel, and restructuring a key defining identity dilemma. For example, later in the therapy process, Marjorie might share a memory that she had suppressed (to survive) of her first partner sexually exploiting her. The therapist again might invite Marjorie to revisit the experience, with attention to the possibility of retraumatizing the client (i.e., carefully considering the client's window of tolerance) and with the clear goal of helping her to feel what was intolerable to feel then but now can in the presence of a supportive other/supportive others. In choreographing this corrective emotional experience (Move 3 of the Tango) with this goal at the forefront, the therapist dims the light and volume on the perpetrator, even blocks access with an imaginary wall or curtain, and instead, focuses on and illuminates the connection between Marjorie and key others. The therapist reminds Marjorie that the therapist is present and that older, wiser Marjorie is, too, and possibly, if made explicit earlier in Stage 1, that her current partner can also be a sensitive and understanding resource, as a safe other to support her in her emotional experience and not as a witness to the details.

Important as well at this stage of the process is level of experiencing. Here we turn again to the work and wisdom of Eugene Gendlin (1981) and the Experiencing Scale developed by Gendlin and his colleagues (Klein et al., 1969). As described earlier and in other writings (Johnson & Campbell, 2022), the Experiencing Scale describes seven levels of depth of client emotional engagement and involvement with ongoing felt experience. Levels 1 to 3 are characterized as "talking about" rather than "feeling into." The client is generally detached from inner experience and there is a low level of emotional engagement. At Level 4 (or above), the desired level of experience in Stage 2, the client begins to turn inward in a process of discovery and exploration, where bodily feelings are made more explicit and attention turns to emotion and thoughts about self. As the experience takes hold, clients can get fully absorbed, signaling the therapist to follow rather than lead in the organic growth process. As the client stays in this absorbed state, fully present, increased self-reflection and curiosity ensue, along with felt shifts. New meanings and heightened awareness emerge, previously implicit feelings become explicit, new perspectives are gained on unsolvable problems, and vision and perspective are expanded, made more vivid, more alive.

While relationally resourcing Marjorie in the context of this defining experience, the therapist encourages and supports a deeper level of experiencing and engagement with emotion, not for the sole purposes of catharsis or having a voice that she might not have had or as a means of desensitization. Rather, the goal, once again, is to accompany Marjorie into the felt experience associated with this key defining identity dilemma, allowing her to feel what was intolerable and unsafe to feel at the time of the event (at a level of experiencing of 4 and above), then providing her with the comfort and support she needed at the time but did not have. For example, the therapist might say, "As you are there in that room, and I'm there, too, at the doorway, can you find and feel you, that older wiser you? Where are you? The therapist ensures and makes explicit resourcing. Assuming Marjorie nods yes, the therapist might say, "Good, and as you find you in that experience and begin to feel some of the terrible feelings you would not have felt safe to feel at the time, what happens next? What are you drawn to do?" Notice there are several options here, but the goal is to keep it generally open-ended, trusting the power and potency of attachment and the foundation that was built in Stage 1. Though a variety of options are possible, what is often the case in circumstances involving key others who are no longer important in the client's life, is escaping, leaving the scene to never return. This is done with newfound confidence and competence, a solution to no-solution vulnerability, and a way out of feeling trapped and helpless. It is at this point that the therapist might then turn to a current resource, such as Marjorie's partner. "Can he comfort you now? Would you allow him to do that?" This can be done imaginally as the session comes to a close and/or as Marjorie moves out of the therapy process and returns to her home and current context. Whatever the case, it is important that this engaged encounter is punctuated by Moves 4 and 5 of the Tango, allowing the client to consolidate the key therapeutic gain(s) that has/have been made, and the therapist to link it explicitly and deliberately to the central aim of Stage 2, restructuring self and system (view of self and other). "As your partner holds you, do you feel held? As he looks into your eyes, what do you see? What do his eyes say about how he sees you? Do you take it in? As he shares that, what do you feel about you?"

Relevant here and a guide for the EFIT therapist is how we understand and work with shame. Once again, the expectation is that shame cannot be fully resolved in the initial stage of therapy, given that it is intrinsically linked with the view of self. As described by Paul Gilbert

(2011), "Shame belongs to a family of emotions that are linked to the very sense of oneself—the kind of person we feel we are . . . how we believe we exist for others . . . and how we exist in our own minds." In Stage 1, the EFIT therapist mentally notes but does not make explicit any shame/negative model of self. Similarly, attention is not drawn to shame/self-loathing. Rather, the EFIT therapist contextualizes and validates shame in the context of prior (and potentially current) experience. For example, the therapist might say, "It makes sense that you would hide, Sierra, shrink and pull away from school, given some of the experiences you described of racism, labeling, and a general sense of isolation within the dominant culture. It makes sense that you shut down, went numb, that was your only recourse as a young child." Recognizing that shame can be viewed on a continuum and/or as multilayered (e.g., early childhood trauma followed by years of substance abuse and betrayal in relationships), in some cases, the therapist can contain and contextualize shame with relative ease, and at other times, shame continually emerges as a barrier through the therapy process. Understood as central to self and self-development and growth in relationship, the therapist might, at times, also highlight the impact on current relationships (e.g., "They cannot see you if you are not to be seen"). Interventions might then be introduced with sensitive attunement to help guide the client forward from behind the wall they built and into felt experience (likely accessed through the body). As these strategies are legitimized and contextualized, engaged encounters (Move 3) might be set up between the young self and the older, wiser self as a means of priming and promoting compassion, the antidote to shame. Pacing will depend on various factors, including history of trauma, but also present circumstances and resources. At times, external resources and stability will need to be fostered prior to engaging in such therapeutic work.

Tracking, validation, and reflection in Stage 1 provides a platform to work with and more directly resolve shame in Stage 2. That is, from a stance of empathy and with an understanding of trauma and its impact. In Stage 2, the therapist provides compassion for the client, particularly the younger, vulnerable self, that part of the self that had to shut down to survive. As the therapist repeatedly provides validations and reflections that help anchor the process and provide the client with context for the previously adaptive coping strategy, the client begins to view self and behavior in a more compassionate light. As the client moves into Stage 2 of the therapeutic process, stabilization and resourcing afford greater access to vulnerability (a broader window of tolerance), as well as access to self and other. As key traumatic incidents that have been instrumental in shaping models of self and other are encountered and resolved, shame dissolves alongside increased self-cohesion and integration, and the client's narrative shifts from helplessness to agency, self-sufficiency to reliance, and self-blame/loathing to self-compassion. Grief naturally emerges as clients begin to experience a felt sense of security with themselves and others. The grief process must be named and honored, allowing the client to grieve what was not (e.g., the childhood they did not have, the loving parent they did not have), and making space for the client to fully embrace what is and what is becoming (i.e., secure attachment).

To summarize, as process consultant and temporary attachment figure, the therapist guides and supports the client to feel in the presence and support of a trusted other(s) what was intolerable to feel during pivotal moments that have been instrumental in shaping view of self and other. This deepens in Stage 2 such that models of self and other are more accessible to revision. The therapist follows and leads. As the client becomes absorbed in experience (at Level 4 and above on the Experiencing Scale), felt shifts occur and the organic process takes hold in deeper and more sustainable ways. These Stage 2 corrective emotional experiences or identity epiphanies expand and change perspective, dissolve shame/self-loathing/blame, lead to self-integration and coherence, broaden view of others, and widen affect regulation capacity in a manner that allows for ongoing growth. By the end of Stage 2, the organic growth process has been kick-started and is well underway.

In short, by the end of Stage 2, the following changes can be anticipated:

- increased awareness of and access to vulnerabilities and needs;
- increased access to self and experience;
- improved capacity to assert and share these needs, vulnerabilities, fears, and longings coherently and directly to key others/attachment figures;
- the gap between trigger and response is broadened, representative also of increased flexibility and adaptability in the face of stress and increased resilience;
- greater capacity to move into and through emotion, and to use it as a compass for life (effective affect regulation);
- indications of increased confidence and competence are noted, along with a sense of belonging;
- capacity to love and be loved, to take in the care, love, and support of another; and
- increased hope for the future and resolving of the past, often described as a "new lease on life."

STAGE 3: CONSOLIDATION

In consolidating therapeutic gains in Stage 3, changes are distilled, highlighted, and celebrated. New action tendencies and increased flexibility are made vivid. Commonly, new solutions to old problems are identified, realized, and implemented. An expanded view of self is exemplified, consolidated, and integrated. New modes of engagement with key others are explored and highlighted. Shifts in the client's narrative are illuminated and the client is invited into a vision of the future with new goals and aspirations.

It is here, as well, that clients might naturally begin to revisit and consider renegotiating relationships with key others (e.g., a previously abusive or neglectful parent). Once again, it is important that the therapist supports and listens, rather than assumes and guides, knowing that the client now has the more positive view of self and coping resources to be their own guide. Key attachment figures who might have been introduced at the outset of therapy as those who have caused harm, might now be seen in a different light, themselves perhaps in a different position in life. Most certainly, the client has a different vantage point, now standing on more solid ground with a bolstered sense of self and increased capacity and agency.

In some cases, the therapy process might be guided by the Attachment Injury Resolution Model (AIRM), advanced and empirically validated in the EFT couple literature (see also Johnson, 2019). The term *attachment injury* was coined to capture the sense of betrayal and mistrust that ensues following significant disappointment during a time of vulnerability/need in couple relationships (e.g., "You weren't there for me when my mother died/when the baby was born/you betrayed me with another partner"). Very often such incidents are accompanied by a resolve to never trust again and are associated with trauma reactions such as insomnia, flashbacks, nightmares, and intrusive memories. We can also apply the term here and the model of resolution. In the case of developmental trauma (e.g., the developing child's sense of self infused with shame and their perceptions of others as unavailable and untrustworthy), once some resolution is gained through psychotherapy, they might then seek additional resolve with key others. From an EFIT/attachment point of view, resolution involves the key other being able to witness and acknowledge the pain of the injured child/adult, that individual (the client) being able to take it in and be soothed by the acknowledgment, and some type of apology/resolve to forge a new relationship must be provided. With this assurance, the client and key other might then begin to cocreate a new narrative together. In other cases, either imaginally in therapy through Move 3 encounters or in their current context, clients might attempt repair and fail, and thereby let go of all hope that they might get the love and care they need and deserve and/or needed and deserved in the past. In such moments of realization, grief is inevitable and must be acknowledged and worked through to make space for something or someone new.

Also in Stage 3, the therapist helps the client prepare for and anticipate possible triggering of symptoms from events such as anniversaries of loss or traumatic incidents, and a potential resurgence in symptoms. In the case of traumatic loss, for example, clients might develop opportunities to proactively prepare and plan for the anniversary of the loss (e.g., organizing family gatherings, planning for a special dinner, or planting a tree). In situations involving likely ongoing exposure to trauma, such as in the case of work with first responders, and/or the probability of continued experiences of racism or discrimination, the therapist might both consolidate gains and further highlight personal resources (and risk factors) with the aim of promoting ongoing resilience.

In the context of couple therapy, we would assert that the goal and expectation is not the absence of conflict, but rather the capacity to regain balance and ability to repair in ways that preserve and even strengthen the relationship. Similarly, in individual therapy, it is not anticipated that clients will never experience symptoms, such as heightened anxiety or low mood, under conditions of stress or conflict. This is especially so when biological factors such as longstanding familial depression are at play or when contextual factors are such that stress remains omnipresent. The assumption is that when clients are fully alive and can move into and through emotion, using it as a guide and compass for life and reach to and respond to key others, they will of course, lose their emotional balance, but also have increased capacity to regain it.

In summary, by the end of Stage 3, the following can be anticipated:

- perception expands beyond threat and danger;
- emotion expands beyond negative affect and clients exhibit increased capacity for effective affect regulation and emotional balance, and the capacity to regain that balance;
- cognition shifts as clients gain increased capacity to move with and through experience, affording possibilities to reflect on, learn, and grow from experience;
- action shifts as clients gain a greater sense of agency and increased flexibility, with increased space between trigger and response;
- relationships move from threat to secure connection as clients gain the ability to tune into themselves and respond to others;
- definition of self is expanded and developed, is integrated and

coherent, and is infused with a sense of confidence and competence, allowing clients to live fully and to continually grow in their most important relationships.

SUMMARY

Dancing the EFIT Tango through the Three-Stage Process: Key Considerations

1. The EFIT Tango is a set of macro interventions repeatedly used to propel the therapeutic process forward. Pacing is guided by the client, and by the therapeutic process. As the therapist tunes into and stays attuned to the client's capacity and various process elements, interventions are introduced and titrated accordingly.

2. For clients with severe trauma histories, little to no reprieve, and few resources, developing trust and sharing their stories (sometimes for the first time) can be very difficult. Gaps in memory and an incoherent narrative are common. Also likely is a longer therapy process, especially in Stage 1, with a focus only on Move 1 of the Tango initially, with the explicit aim of building trust, awareness, and coherence.

3. As a mirror (Move 1) is put up for clients in these early sessions in Stage 1, clients begin to see themselves, and ideally, start to develop some self-compassion. As importantly, they feel seen and heard.

4. The EFIT Tango can be used to help clients access and engage with key others or experiences (e.g., experiences of competence such as that found in sport, writing, art, or music and/or islands of security with key others) as a means of resourcing the client.

5. Clients with a less severe trauma history and/or greater personal and/or social resources are often able to move into frightening, alien, and unacceptable emotion more readily than those with more limited resources and restrictive strategies. Once again, sensitive attunement guides pacing. In some cases, affect assembly occurs with ease, in others, more time and care are required. In the former case, following an effective Move 1 reflection, the therapist can often help organize and order emotion through further accurate reflection, then more directly guide the client into deepening (Move 2), followed by Moves 3, 4, and 5. In the latter case, it may take time (even more than one session) to help clients tune into and assemble, order and organize their experience, allowing for more coherence and clarity to then move toward deepening and into Moves 3 through 5 of the Tango.

6. For some clients, after formal affect assembly, this awareness of the key elements of emotion can be readily built upon in future sessions, with the therapist guiding the client into deepening with relative ease. In such circumstances, a return to ordering emotion and creating a more coherent narrative is not necessary. Rather, various doorways (i.e., key pivotal events that have shaped model of self and other) into frightening, alien, and unacceptable emotion (Move 2) can be opened and corrective emotional experiences (Move 3) choreographed.

7. The EFIT Tango is intended to be used fluidly and flexibly as the therapist guides and accompanies, follows and leads. At times, for example, following a Move 3 encounter when blocks to receiving love and care are identified in Move 4, the therapist might then return to Move 3 as a means of attempting to reach deeper levels of engagement and increased risk to trust and more fully engage.

8. As clients move through Stage 1 and into Stage 2 with increased capacity (i.e., more emotional balance, a wider gap between trigger and response, increased flexibility, a broader window of tolerance and greater ease in moving to their leading edge), Tango interventions can be pitched at a deeper level, with the expectation that clients will be able to move more deeply into core vulnerabilities (Move 2) and stay at deeper levels of experiencing for longer periods. As the flow of the therapeutic process takes hold in Stage 2 and clients are absorbed at deeper levels of experience, the therapist can, at times, be less active in blocking exits, follow more than lead, and rely on the power of attachment and the now stronger, wiser, more emotionally balanced client (e.g., as the younger self enters a difficult scene or encounters core vulnerability, the adult self might be asked, "What are you drawn to do?"). At other times, despite moving into Stage 2, the propensity remains in the direction of protective strategies, and it is important that the therapist continue to focus the session, blocking detours or more intellectual discussions, providing more support and rationale, and/or accessing resources, and thereby encouraging deeper levels of engagement for longer periods.

9. As the frightening becomes manageable, the alien becomes familiar, and the unacceptable becomes tolerable as clients move through Stage 1 and into Stage 2, the platform is built for clients to enter into, embody, and face the core vulnerabilities and dilemmas that have imprisoned them more explicitly and directly. With fundamental definitions of self and other now more available and open to modification, Move 3 encounters are more explicitly aimed at engaging with core defining experiences and vulnerabilities, and Move 4 is explicitly aimed at exploring the restructuring of self and system. For example, as the

client begins to reveal shifts in model of self, the therapist might ask, "When you see you, what do you see?" or "What might your partner (or another key attachment figure) say about what is different and what is the same, relative to the outset of therapy?"

10. In Stage 3, it is often helpful to return to inquiries about trigger and response, perception, bodily sense and meaning making as a means of comparing then and now, and highlighting the possibility of returning to habitual strategies under conditions of stress, threat, or new trauma, and how best to ensure a timely return to emotional balance and to continued growth and resilience.

KEY TAKEAWAYS

Anticipated Outcomes toward the End of Stage 1 in EFIT

- Increased awareness of patterns of strategies for managing stress (i.e., action tendencies) and interactions with key others.
- A more coherent narrative, more linked to symptoms and to the way client defines self and others.
- Improved emotional balance/wider window of tolerance (more flexibility, less numbing/reactivity, greater capacity to move into and through emotion).
- A reduction in symptoms (e.g., anxiety, depression, intrusive symptoms such as flashbacks, nightmares, irritability, and anger).
- Increased awareness of fears, longings, vulnerabilities, and their legitimacy.
- Improved exploration (Accessibility/Openness, Responsiveness, and Engagement) with self and key others; more discovery-oriented.
- Movement toward more self- and other-acceptance and compassion.
- Increased access to key elements of models of self and other, and increased flexibility.
- New sense of hope and self-efficacy.

Anticipated Outcomes toward the End of Stage 2 in EFIT

- Increased awareness of and access to vulnerabilities and needs.
- Increased access to self and experience.
- Improved capacity to assert and share these needs, vulnerabilities, fears, and longings coherently and directly to key others/ attachment figures.

▪ The gap between trigger and response is broadened, representative also of increased flexibility and adaptability in the face of stress— increased resilience.

▪ Greater capacity to move into and through emotion and use it as a compass for life (effective affect regulation).

▪ Indications of increased confidence and competence are noted, along with sense of belonging.

▪ Capacity to love and be loved, and take in the care, love, and support of another.

▪ Increased hope for the future and resolve of the past, often described as a "new lease on life."

Anticipated Outcomes as Clients Move through Stage 3 in EFIT

▪ Perception expands beyond threat and danger.

▪ Emotion expands beyond negative affect and clients exhibit increased capacity for effective affect regulation and emotional balance, and the capacity to regain that balance.

▪ Cognition shifts as clients gain increased capacity to move with and through experience, affording possibilities to reflect on, learn, and grow from experience.

▪ Action shifts as clients gain a greater sense of agency and increased flexibility, with increased space between trigger and response.

▪ Relationships move from threat to secure connection as clients gain the ability to tune into themselves and respond to others.

▪ Definition of self is expanded and developed, is integrated and coherent, and infused with a sense of confidence and competence, allowing clients to live fully and to continually grow in their most important relationships.

References

Allan, R., Edwards, C., & Lee, N. (2022). Cultural adaptations of emotionally focused therapy. *Journal of Couple & Relationship Therapy, 22*(1), 43–63.

Anderson, R. (1974). Notes of a survivor. In S. Troup & W. Greene (Eds.), *The patient, death, and the family* (pp. 71–82). Scribner.

Arnold, M. B. (1960). *Emotion and personality.* Columbia University Press.

Averill, L. A., Averill, C. L., Pietrzak, R. H., Charney, D. S., & Southwick, S. M. (2021). Psychoneurobiology of resilience. In M. J. Friedman, P. P. Schnurr, & T. M. Keane (Eds.), *Handbook of PTSD: Science and practice* (pp. 551–569). Guilford Press.

Barlow, D. H., Allen, L. B., & Choate, M. L. (2004). Toward a unified treatment for emotional disorders. *Behavioral Therapy, 35,* 205–230.

Barlow, D. H., Farshione, T., Fairholme, C., Ellard, K., Boisseau, C., Allen, L., . . . Cassiello-Robbins, C. (2011). *Unified protocol for transdiagnostic treatment of emotional disorders.* Oxford University Press.

Bonanno, G. A. (2004). Loss, trauma, and human resilience: Have we underestimated the human capacity to thrive after extremely aversive events? *American Psychologist, 59*(1), 20–28.

Bonanno, G. A. (2019). *The other side of sadness: What the new science of bereavement tells us about life after loss.* Basic Books.

Bonanno, G. A., Galea, S., Bucciarelli, A., & Vlahov, D. (2006). Psychological resilience after disaster: New York City in the aftermath of the September 11th terrorist attack. *Psychological Science, 17*(3), 181–186.

Bonanno, G. A., Westphal, M., & Mancini, A. D. (2011). Resilience to loss and potential trauma. *Annual Review of Clinical Psychology, 7,* 511–535.

Bowlby, J. (1980). *Attachment and loss: Vol. 3. Loss: Sadness and depression.* Basic Books.

Bradley, B., & Furrow, J. L. (2004). Toward a mini-theory of the blamer softening event: Tracking the moment-by-moment process. *Journal of Marital and Family Therapy, 30*(2), 233–246.

Bradley, B., & Furrow, J. (2007). Inside blamer softening: Maps and missteps. *Journal of Systemic Therapies, 26*(4), 25–43.

Briere, J. (2011). *Trauma symptom inventory (TSI-2) professional manual* (2nd ed.). Psychological Assessment Resources.

Burgess Moser, M. (2012). *The cognitive-affective and behavioural impact of emotionally focused couple therapy* [Doctoral dissertation, Université d'Ottawa/University of Ottawa]. Library and Archives Canada.

Burgess Moser, M., Johnson, S. M., Dalgleish, T. L., Wiebe, S. A., & Tasca, G. (2017). The impact of blamer-softening on romantic attachment in emotionally focused couples therapy. *Journal of Marital and Family Therapy, 44*(4), 640–654.

Chodron, P. (2002). *Comfortable with uncertainty: 108 teachings.* Shambhala.

Dalgleish, T. L., Johnson, S. M., Burgess Moser, M., Wiebe, S. A., & Tasca, G. A. (2015). Predicting key change events in emotionally focused couple therapy. *Journal of Marital and Family Therapy, 41*(3), 260–275.

Damasio, A. (1999). *The feeling of what happens: Body and emotion in the making of consciousness.* Harcourt.

Davis, D. E., DeBlaere, C., Hook, J. N., Choe, E., Worthington, E. L., Owen, J., . . . Placers, V. (2018). The multicultural orientation framework: A narrative review. *Psychotherapy, 55* (1), 89–100.

Didion, J. (2007). *The year of magical thinking.* Vintage.

Eisenberger, N. I., & Lieberman, M. D. (2004). Why rejection hurts: A common neural alarm system for physical and social pain. *Trends in Cognitive Sciences, 8*(7), 294–300.

Eisenberger, N. I., Lieberman, M. D., & Williams, K. D. (2003). Does rejection hurt? An FMRI study of social exclusion. *Science, 302*(5643), 290–292.

Fairbairn, W. R. D. (1952). *An object relations theory of the personality.* Basic Books.

Feeney, B. C. (2004). A secure base: Responsive support of goal strivings and exploration in adult intimate relationships. *Journal of Personality and Social Psychology, 87*(5), 631–648.

Felitti, V. J., Anda, R. F., Nordenberg, D., Williamson, D. F., Spitz, A. M., Edwards, . . . Marks, J. S. (1998). Relationship of childhood abuse and household dysfunction to many of the leading causes of death in adults: The Adverse Childhood Experiences (ACE) study. *American Journal of Preventative Medicine, 14*(4), 245–258.

Fraley, R. C., Fazzari, D. A., Bonanno, G. A., & Dekel, S. (2006). Attachment and psychological adaptation in high exposure survivors of the September 11th attack on the World Trade Center. *Personality and Social Psychology Bulletin, 32*(4), 538–551.

Friedman, M. J., Schnurr, P. P., & Keane, T. M. (2021). *The handbook of PTSD: Science and practice.* Guilford Press.

Gendlin, E. T. (1996). *Focusing-oriented psychotherapy: A manual of the experiential method.* Guilford Press.

Goldstein, J. (1993). *Insight meditation.* Shambala.

Guillory, P. T. (2022). *Emotionally focused therapy with African American couples: Love heals.* Routledge.

Haidt, J. (2023, February 22). *Social media is a major cause of the mental illness epidemic in teen girls: Here's the evidence.* After Babel. *www.afterbabel.com/p/social-media-mental-illness-epidemic*

Halchuk, R., Makinen, J. & Johnson, S. M. (2010). Resolving attachment injuries in couples using emotionally focused therapy: A 3-year follow-up. *Journal of Couple and Relationship Therapy, 9*(1), 31–47.

Hayes, L., & Allan, R. (2024). EFT for three: Working with polyamorous relationships. *The Family Journal, 32*(3), 346–353.

Herman, J. L. (1992). *Trauma and recovery.* Basic Books.

Holt-Lunstad, J., Smith, T. B., Baker, M., Harris, T., & Stephenson, D. (2015). Loneliness and social isolation as risk factors for mortality: A meta-analytic review. *Perspectives on Psychological Science, 10*(2), 227–237.

Johnson, S. M. (1986). Bonds or bargains: Relationship paradigms and their significance for marital therapy. *Journal of Marital and Family Therapy, 12*(3), 259–267.

Johnson, S. M. (2002). *Emotionally focused couple therapy with trauma survivors: Strengthening attachment bonds.* Guilford Press.

Johnson, S. M. (2008). *Hold me tight: Seven conversations for a lifetime of love.* Little, Brown.

Johnson, S. M. (2013). *Love sense: The revolutionary new science of romantic relationships.* Little, Brown.

Johnson, S. M. (2019). *Attachment theory in practice: Emotionally focused therapy (EFT) with individuals, couples, and families.* Guilford Press.

Johnson, S. M. (2020). *The practice of emotionally focused couple therapy: Creating connection* (3rd ed. rev.). Routledge.

Johnson, S. M. (2022). *Edgar & Elouise.* Friesen Press.

Johnson, S. M., Burgess Moser, M., Beckes, L., Smith, A., Dalgleish, T., Halchuk, R., . . . Coan, J. A. (2013). Soothing the threatened brain: Leveraging contact comfort with emotionally focused therapy. *PLOS ONE, 8*(11): e79314.

Johnson, S, M., & Campbell, T. L. (2022). *A primer for emotionally focused individual therapy (EFIT): Cultivating fitness and growth in every client.* Routledge.

Johnson, S. M., Makinen, J., & Millikin, J. (2001). Attachment injuries in couple relationships: A new perspective on impasses in couples therapy. *Journal of Marital and Family Therapy, 27*(2), 145–155.

Kabat-Zinn, J. (2003). Mindfulness-based stress reduction. *Constructivism in the Human Sciences, 8*(2), 73–107.

Kabat-Zinn, J. (2023). *Wherever you go, there you are: Mindfulness meditation in everyday life.* Hachette.

Kailanko, S., Wiebe, S. A., Tasca, G. A., & Laitila, A. A. (2022). Somatic interventions and depth of experiencing in emotionally focused couple therapy. *International Journal of Systemic Therapy, 33*(2), 109–128.

Karakurt, G. & Keiley, M. (2009). Integration of a cultural lens with emotionally focused therapy. *Journal of Couple and Relationship Therapy, 8*, 4–14.

Kazda, L., McGeechan, K., Bell, K., Thomas, R., & Barratt, A. (2022).

Association of attention-feficit/hyperactivity disorder diagnosis with adolescent quality of life. *JAMA Netw Open, 5*(10), Article e2236364.

Kehle-Forbes, S. M., Meis, L. A., Polusny, M. A., & Spoont, M. R. (2015). Treatment initiation and dropout from prolonged exposure and cognitive processing therapy in a VA outpatient clinic. *Psychological Trauma: Theory, Research, Practice, and Policy, 8*(1), 107–114.

Klein, M. H., Mathiew, P. L., Gendlin, E. T., & Kiesler, D. J. (1969). *The Experiencing Scale: A research and training manual* (Vol.1). Wisconsin Psychiatric Institute.

Knobloch, L. K., & Owens, J. L. (2024). Moral injury among first responders: Experience, effects, and advice in their own words. *Psychological Services, 21*(3), 500–508.

Linhoff, A. Y., & Allan, R. (2019). A narrative expansion of emotionally focused therapy with intercultural couples. *The Family Journal, 27*(1), 44–49.

Lutkenhaus, P., Grossman, K. E., & Grossman, K. (1985). Infant mother attachment at twelve months and style of interaction with a stranger at the age of three years. *Child Development, 56*(6), 1538–1542.

Makinen, J., & Johnson, S. M. (2006). Resolving attachment injuries in couples using EFT: Steps towards forgiveness and reconciliation. *Journal of Consulting and Clinical Psychology, 74*(6), 1055–1064.

Mesquita, B. (2022). *Between us: How cultures create emotions.* Norton.

Mesquita, B., & Walker, R. (2002). Cultural differences in emotions: A context for interpreting emotional experiences. *Behaviour Research and Therapy, 41*, 777–793.

Mikulincer, M., Florian, V., & Weller, A. (1993). Attachment styles, coping strategies and posttraumatic psychological stress: The impact of the Gulf War in Israel. *Journal of Personality and Social Psychology, 64*, 817–826.

Mikulincer, M., & Shaver, P. R. (2004). Security-based self-representations in adulthood: Contents and processes. In W. S. Rholes & J. A. Simpson (Eds.), *Adult attachment: Theory, research, and clinical implications* (pp. 159–195). Academic Press.

Mikulincer, M., & Shaver, P. R. (2013). Attachment insecurities and disordered patterns of grief. In M. Stroebe, H. J. Schut, P. Boelen, & J. van den Bout (Eds.), *Complicated grief: Scientific foundations for health care professionals* (pp. 190–213). Routledge.

Mikulincer, M., & Shaver, P. R. (2023). *Attachment theory applied: Fostering personal growth through healthy relationships.* Guilford Press.

Mikulincer, M., Shaver, P. R., & Horesh, N. (2006). Attachment bases of emotion regulation and posttraumatic adjustment. In D. K. Snyder, J. A. Simpson, & J. N. Hughes (Eds.), *Emotion regulation in families: Pathways to dysfunction and health* (pp. 77–99). American Psychological Association.

Mowrer, O. H. (1960). *Learning theory and behavior.* Wiley.

Myung, H. S., Furrow, J. L., & Lee, N. A. (2022). Understanding the emotional landscape in the withdrawer re-engagement and blamer softening EFCT change events. *Journal of Marital and Family Therapy, 48*(3), 758–776.

Naaman, S., Pappas, J. D., Makinen, J., Zuccarini, D., & Johnson-Douglas, S. M. (2005). Treating attachment injured couples with emotionally focused therapy: A case study approach. *Psychiatry: Interpersonal and Biological Processes, 68*(1), 55–77.

Nightingale, M., Awosan, C. I., & Stavrianopoulos, K. (2019). Emotionally focused therapy: A culturally sensitive approach for African American heterosexual couples. *Journal of Family Psychotherapy, 30*(3), 221–244.

Perry, B. D. & Winfrey, O. (2021). *What happened to you? Conversations on trauma, resilience, and healing.* Flatiron Books.

Petty-John, M. E., Tseng, C-F., & Blow, A. J. (2020). Therapeutic utility of discussing therapist/client intersectionality in treatment: When and how? *Family Process, 59*(2), 313–327.

Porges, S. W. (2011). *The polyvagal theory: Neurophysiological foundations of emotion, attachment, communication and self-regulation.* Norton.

Rogers, C. (1961). *On becoming a person.* Houghton Mifflin.

Rosenbaum, R. & Bohart, A. (2021). Mindfulness is full engagement. *The Humanistic Psychologist, 49*(1), 122–132.

Spengler, P. M., Lee, N. A., Wiebe, S. A., & Wittenborn, A. K. (2024). A comprehensive meta-analysis on the efficacy of emotionally focused couple therapy. *Couple and Family Psychology: Research and Practice, 13*(2), 81–99.

Strathearn, L., Giannotti, M., Mills, R., Kisely, S., Najman, J., & Abajobir, A. (2020). Long-term cognitive, psychological, and health outcomes associated with childhood abuse and neglect. *Pediatrics, 146*(4), Article e20200438.

Tedeschi, R. G., & Calhoun, L. G. (1995). *Trauma and transformation: Growth in the aftermath of suffering.* SAGE.

Teicher, M. H., & Samson, J. A. (2016). Annual research review: Enduring neurobiological effects of childhood abuse and neglect. *Journal of Child Psychiatry, 57*(3), 241–266.

van der Kolk, B. (2015). *The body keeps the score.* Penguin Books.

Wiebe, S., Johnson, S. M., Allan, R., Campbell, T. L., Greenman, P. S., Fairweather, D. R., . . . Tasca, G. A. (2025). A randomized controlled trial of emotionally focused individual therapy (EFIT) for depression and anxiety. *Psychotherapy.* [Advance online publication]

Yalom, I. D. (1980). *Existential psychotherapy.* Basic Books.

Zuccarini, D. J., Johnson, S. M., Dalgleish, T., & Makinen, J. (2013). Forgiveness and reconciliation in emotionally focused therapy for couples: The client change process and therapist interventions. *Journal of Marriage and Family Therapy, 39*(2), 148–162.

Index

Note. f following a page number indicates a figure.

Abandonment and rejection, fear of, 3,
    23, 28, 139
  attachment science and, 24, 31
  EFT Tango and, 48
  isolation and loneliness, 27
  Marjorie case example, 223, 224
  Randy and Karen case example, 146,
    149
  Sierra case example, 87, 88
Ability to explore and learn, principle of
    attachment, 23
Accessibility, Responsiveness, and
    Engagement (ARE), 17, 135
  as attachment principle, 22–23
  presence for collaborative therapy
    relationship, 54, 68
  in sense of self, 19
Accurate and on-target reflections, in
    PACE, 76–77, 105
Addiction, 4, 82, 146, 152
Adult attachment
  anxious attachment, anger and
    demanding, 24
  avoidant attachment, reluctance for
    connection, 24
  brain scan research, 17–18
  disorganized attachment, paradoxical
    style of, 25
  Shaver and Mikulincer on, 17
Affecting assembly and deepening, Move
    2 of EFIT Tango, 35, 135
  assembling elements of emotion, 40–41
  body sensation that goes with trigger,
    41, 87

core emotion, reorganization of self,
    43
emotion colors perception and mean
    making, 43
emotion communication and
    motivation, 43
emotional handles of client, 42–43
finding action impulse that emotion
    elicits, 42
finding cognition/meaning that goes
    with trigger and sensation, 41, 87
integrates elements of emotion,
    trigger, perception, body sensation,
    cognition and action impulse
    together, 42, 87
reflects and repeats trigger, sensation,
    and meaning, 41, 87
Saul case example, 119, 123
Sierra case example, 81, 87, 92
therapist focuses on tracking emotion,
    39–40
Agency, lack of, 6–7, 151
  emotional isolation and, 21, 41, 56
AIRM. *See* Attachment Injury Resolution
    Model
Alexander, Franz, 8
American Psychiatric Association DSM-
    5-TR, 6
Anger, 10, 87, 107, 168, 205, 207–208
  anxious attachment and, 24
  core emotion of, 40, 214
  as prototypical way of coping, 72, 79
  reactive, 78, 136
  validation of, 78–79

Anxious attachment
  anger and demanding behavior, 24
  insensitive parenting and early
    separation as cause of, 24
Anxious dismissing attachment, 23
ARE. *See* Accessibility, Responsiveness,
  and Engagement
Assessment as guide through three stages
  of EFIT intervention, 70. *See also*
  Sierra case example
  attachment security as benchmark, 71,
    104
  attachment understanding of potential
    trauma impacts, 71–72, 104
  client strengths and resources
    illuminated, 80–81, 105
  developmental frame guides
    understanding, pacing, intervention,
    72, 104
  focus on present process, 74, 104
  nonpathologizing approach of EFT,
    72–73, 104
  ongoing assessment guiding
    intervention, 79–80, 105
  PACE in therapeutic process, 105
  safety established and maintained with
    PACE, 76–77, 105
  surface symptoms and underlying
    attachment security, 74, 104
  therapist focus with CARE, 74–75, 104
Attachment, in CARE, 75
Attachment injury, 230
Attachment Injury Resolution Model
  (AIRM), 138–139, 172–173, 230
Attachment map, to core emotions, 29,
  32, 98
Attachment principles, 31
  ability to explore and learn, 23
  ARE, 22–23
  safe haven, 21–22, 27, 70, 141, 151,
    204
  secure base, 22
Attachment science
  abandonment and rejection, fear of,
    24, 31
  capacity, 71, 75, 140
  change possibility, 26
  common impacts of trauma, 31–32
  constructive dependency on others, 19
  down-to-earth perspective, 26–30
  dysfunctional responses, trauma trap, 2
  framework for core structure of shared
    humanity, 20–21
  healing guided by, 18

  as healing path, 15–32
  image of health, 71
  interdependent rational beings, 18–29
  key points of, 31–32
  role of emotions, 18
  Shaver and Mikulincer on adult
    attachment, 17
  traumatic experiences through lens of,
    13, 217
  on true healing and frozen state, 19
  understanding fear with, 12
Attachment security, 71, 74, 104
Attachment theory, of Bowlby
  anxious dismissing attachment, 23
  avoidant attachment, 24
  disorganized attachment, 25
  secure attachment, 23, 50, 72, 145,
    175, 198, 199
  on social bonding, 16
  on trauma of emotional isolation, 16
Attachment Theory in Practice (Johnson),
  129
Avoidant attachment strategy
  adult reluctance for connection, 24
  emotional absence or indifference,
    24

B

Barlow, David, 8
Bertalanffy, Ludwig von, 5
Blocks, 221
  to connection, 135–136, 172
  to growth, 71, 73, 80
  identification of, to mobilize grief,
    214–215
  Move 3 of EFIT Tango, 44, 51, 233
  Move 4 of EFIT Tango, 47
  process of moving from, 55–56
  trauma and emotion, 206
The Body Keeps the Score (van der Kolk),
  3, 222
Bonanno, George, 209
Bonding
  Bowlby on mother with child, 17
  conversations in EFCT, 26
Bowlby, John, 131
  on bonding process of mother with
    child, 17
  on depression, 28, 73
  on experiences of loss and separation,
    15
  focus on mother and child interaction,
    16–17

on impact of separateness and
connection, 15
London Child Guidance Clinic, 16
on negative emotional disorders of
anxiety and depression, 73
Tavistock Clinic research, 16
Brain scan research on adult attachment,
17–18

C

Campbell, T. Leanne, 134
Capacity, 134, 139, 173, 208, 223–224,
231, 234–235
attachment and, 71, 75, 140
first responder variable, 218
flexibility and, 140, 142, 144, 174, 219
increased security and, 73, 143
PACE pacing process with attention to,
76, 77, 105
regulation, 229
relational, 147, 151, 157
rigidity and limited, 72
Saul case example, 123
Sierra case example, 85, 86, 89, 92,
94–95, 97
window of tolerance, 51, 75, 80, 89,
92, 94, 123, 199
Yezda case example, 175, 176, 179,
180–181
CARE. *See* Context, Attachment,
Relationship and Emotion
CBT. *See* Cognitive-behavioral therapy
Change
attachment science on possibility of, 26
Bertalanffy on levels of, 5
Didion on, 210–211
EFT stage 2 on deepened level of
flexibility, 142
first- and second-level, 5
Kessler on loss and, 210
Move 4 of EFIT Tango, 46
Move 5 in EFIT Tango, 48
traumatic experiences and self and
world engagement, 2
traumatic loss, 210–211, 218
Choreographing engaged encounters
with self and other, Move 3 of EFIT
Tango, 46
acceptance and validation, blocks tend
to dissolve, 44, 51, 233
develops core corrective emotional
experience, 44
drama with attachment figure or key
part of self, 43–44

encouragement of clear client statement
of core emotion, 44
FACES, 51
Randy and Karen case example, 162
reflecting, tracking unfolding drama,
66–67
Saul case example, 114, 122–123,
127–128, 131
search for positive resource moments,
45
Sierra case example, 81, 91–93, 95,
99–100
Cognitive-behavioral therapy (CBT), 7
Cognitive processing therapy (CPT), 7
Cognitive reappraisal, 8
Collaborative process, 76
in PACE, 77–78, 105
Stage 1 stabilization, transparency and,
134
therapy relationship, ARE presence,
54, 68
Communication
couple therapy, 27
Move 2 of EFIT Tango, 43
Compassion
as antidote to shame, 127, 142, 162,
170, 173
for self and others, 175
Complex trauma, 3
Connection. *See also* Secure connection
adult avoidant attachment, reluctance
for, 24
blocks to, 135–136, 172
Bowlby on separateness, 15
disorganized attachment, paradoxical,
25
to dissolve shame in EFT stage 2,
135–172
emotional, 21, 26, 204
mental health and loss of social, 29–30
Move 1 of EFIT Tango, 38–39
Waal on human, 17
Consolidation, stage 3 in EFT, 59–60,
69, 220
anticipated outcomes, 231–232, 235
highlighting client narrative shifts,
190–191, 196
Marjorie case example, 230–232
new action and increased flexibility in
response to stress, 187, 196
new solutions identified, 184, 196
shifts in view of engagement and
others, 182, 184–186, 190, 193–194,
196

Consolidation, stage 3 in EFT (*continued*)
　shifts in view of self, 181, 183, 192,
　　196
　therapeutic gains highlighted,
　　celebrated, 181, 187, 190, 196
　Yezda case example, 174–195
Context, Attachment, Relationship and
　Emotion (CARE), 174
　attachment, 75
　building on felt security with, 196
　context in, 74–75
　emotions in, 76
　relationship in, 76
　therapist focus with CARE, 74–75, 104
Context, in CARE, 74–75
Core emotions
　of anger, joy, surprise, sadness, shame
　　and fear, 40, 214
　attachment map to, 29, 32, 98
　Move 2 EFIT Tango, 43
　Move 3 EFIT Tango, 44
Corrective emotional experiences
　Alexander on, 8
　author on need for, 9
　Paula case example, 9–11
Couple therapy
　case example, 147–171
　EFIT stage 2 restructuring, 145–173
　first responder trauma and, 201
　problem solving, communication skills,
　　27
　shaping secure connection in EFCT,
　　27
CPT. *See* Cognitive processing therapy
Cumulative trauma, first responder
　trauma and, 198, 199–200

D

Depression
　Bowlby on, 28, 73
　negative emotional disorder of, 73
　youth and electronic device use, 30
Development
　frame of understanding, 72, 104
　shame and early cumulative
　　experiences, 137–138, 149, 152–153,
　　157, 172
Developmental trauma, 3
Didion, Joan, 210–211
Disorganized attachment, 25
Disorientation, 166
Dissociation, PTSD and survival strategy
　of, 28–29

Down-to-earth perspective, attachment
　science and, 26–30
Drama
　Move 3 of EFIT Tango with attachment
　　figure, 43–44
　reflecting and tracking of unfolding,
　　66–67
　relational, 2
　Saul case example of identity, 129

E

Early cumulative experiences thwart
　development, shame and, 137–138,
　　149, 152–153, 157, 172
Edgar & Elouise (Johnson), 21
EFCT. *See* Emotionally focused therapy
　for couples
EFFT. *See* Emotionally focused therapy
　for families
EFIT. *See* Emotionally focused therapy
　for individuals
EFIT Tango, five macro interventions, 34,
　35*f*, 80
　key points on, 50–51, 232–234
　Move 1 reflecting present process, 35,
　　38–39, 81, 86, 87, 88–89, 98, 112,
　　135
　Move 2 affect assembly and deepening,
　　35, 39–43, 81, 87, 92, 119, 123,
　　135
　Move 3 choreographing engaged
　　encounters with self and others, 35,
　　43–46, 51, 81, 91–93, 94, 99–100,
　　114, 122–123, 127–128, 131, 135,
　　233
　Move 4 processing encounters, 35,
　　46–47, 91, 94, 99, 126, 135, 163
　Move 5 integration and validation, 35,
　　47–48, 93, 94, 122, 128, 132, 170,
　　220
　preparation for, 37–38, 51
EFT. *See* Emotionally focused therapy
Electronic device use, depression and
　suicidality in youth, 30
EMDR. *See* Eye movement desensitization
　and reprocessing therapy
Emotional connection, 21, 26, 204
Emotional handles, in EFT, 42–43, 61,
　76, 116, 119, 121, 139
Emotionally focused therapy (EFT). *See
　also* Consolidation in EFT stage
　3; Restructuring in EFT stage 2;
　Stabilization in EFT stage 1

assessment and intervention through
EFT three-stage process, 81–103
bonding events, 17
emotional handles, 42–43, 61, 76, 116,
119, 121, 139
five Ps, 68
Soft, Slow, Simple, and Specific,
67
transforming trauma with, 1–14
Emotionally focused therapy for couples
(EFCT), 6, 34
ARE presence between partners, 17, 19,
22–23, 54, 68, 135
bonding conversations, 26
softenings, bonding events, 17
trust and access build, 143
Emotionally focused therapy for families
(EFFT), 34
Emotionally focused therapy for
individuals (EFIT), 6, 34. See also
EFIT Tango
addressing types of trauma with,
197–218
Marjorie case example, 219–232
Emotion regulation
Move 1 of EFIT Tango,, 39
as protective factor against effects of
trauma, 4
trauma and limited options for, 23
Emotion
attachment science on impact of, 18
in CARE, 76
EFIT on process of, 40
lead client into and through, 134
Matisse and Mowrer on, 18
Move 2 of EFIT on, 42–43
Saul case example, 111, 117–119
self and experience linked with, 140,
173
Sierra case example, 86–96
as source of growth, 18
trauma blocking of, 206
triggers and elements of, 40–41
working distance from, 65
Empathic attunement and therapist
presence, in PACE, 77, 78, 105
Empathic reflection, in therapy, 2, 78,
105
Evocative imagery or metaphor to capture
meaning, micro intervention of EFT,
65, 69, 108
Evocative questions, micro intervention of
EFT, 38, 62, 65, 69
Existential focus, 3

Experiencing Scale, 142–143
Eye movement desensitization and
reprocessing therapy (EMDR), 7

F

FACES. See Frame, Anticipate, Care,
Engage, Stay
Fear. See also Abandonment and
rejection, fear of
attachment science understanding of,
12
as core emotion, 40, 214
of isolation, 3, 27
Move 4 of EFIT Tango,
acknowledgement of, 47
First-level change, 5
First responder trauma, 204
capacity variable for, 218
CARE and, 197–199
couple therapy, 201
cumulative trauma, 198, 199–200
police officer, 198–199
risk factors, concurrent factors, family
factors for, 197–198
risk of moral injury or distress,
202–203
secure attachment and, 198, 199
self-blame with, 203
substance misuse for coping, 198
work culture, protective factors for,
198
Five Ps in EFT, 56, 68
Flee or freeze response, 208
Flexibility
capacity and, 140, 142, 144, 174, 219
shift from rigidity to, 142, 146, 153,
158–159, 165, 170
stage 3 consolidation, increased, 187,
196
Frame, Anticipate, Care, Engage, Stay
(FACES), in choreographing engaged
encounter, Move 3 of EFIT Tango,
51
Friedman, M. J., 7
Frozen state, 19

G

Grief, 175–176
acknowledgement and honoring of,
with CARE, 196
Bonanno on, 209
identification of blocks to mobilize,
214–215

Grief (*continued*)
  Kessler on loss and change, 210
  shame and sense of loss, 167–168, 173
  traumatic loss and, 211–216, 218
Growth
  blocks to, 71, 73, 80
  client capacity for, 14, 53, 68, 139
  corrective emotional experiences
    fostering, 58–59, 68
  emotions as source of, 18
  posttraumatic, 33

H

Haidt, Jonathon, 29
Handbook of PTSD (Friedman), 7
Healing from trauma. *See also* Trauma,
    assumptions for healing from
  attachment science as path to, 15–32
  attachment science guiding of, 18
Helplessness and lack of agency, 6–7,
    151
  emotional isolation and, 21, 41, 56
Human connection, Waal on, 17

I

Identity
  disturbance in, 7
  epiphanies, 143
  implications in relationship, 20
Inhibitor, shame as, 135, 155, 172
Integration and validation, Move 5 of
    EFIT Tango, 35, 220
  client progress reflection, 47–48
  Randy and Karen case example, 170
  Saul case example, 122, 128, 132
  Sierra case example, 93, 94
Interpretation, micro intervention of EFT,
    63–64, 69
Isolation and loneliness, 3, 6, 23, 25, 63,
    68, 129, 199, 228
  abandonment and rejection, fear of,
    27
  helplessness and emptiness from, 21,
    41, 56
  impact of, 16, 48
  Saul case example, 110, 112–114,
    116–117, 130

J

Janet, Pierre, 4
Johnson, Sue (Susan M.), 18, 21, 129, 134

K

Key points
  of attachment science, 31–32
  of EFIT Tango, 50–51, 232–234
Kolk, Bessel van der, 2–3
Kornfield, Jack, 1

L

Labels and stigma, of trauma survivors,
    28
Life is trouble, Kornfield on, 1
London Child Guidance Clinic, Bowlby
    and, 16
Love Sense (Johnson), 18

M

Macro interventions of EFT, 33, 50–51
  EFT Tango moves, 34–48, 35*f*
  positive outcomes, 34
Marjorie case example, 219–232
Matisse, Henri, 18
Meaning making, 6
Mental health
  constructive dependency as key to, 19
  loss of social connection and, 29–30
  sense of security and, 23
Mental health professionals, 1–2, 20
Micro interventions of EFT, 52
  deepening engagement, 64–65
  evocative imagery or metaphor, 65, 69,
    108
  evocative questions, 38, 62, 65, 69
  interpretation, 63–64, 69
  proxy voice, use of, 65, 69
  reflection, 60–62, 64–65, 69
  reframing, 66, 69
  validation, 62–63, 69, 141–142, 161
Mikulincer, Mario, 17
Mindfulness, 5, 52
Moral injury of distress
  with first responder trauma, 202–203
  survival guilt or, 137
Move 1 of EFIT Tango. *See* Reflecting
    present processes, Move 1 of EFIT
    Tango
Move 2 of EFIT Tango. *See* Affecting
    assembly and deepening, Move 2 of
    EFIT Tango
Move 3 of EFIT Tango. *See*
    Choreographing engaged encounters
    with self and other, Move 3 of EFIT
    Tango

Move 4 of EFIT Tango. *See* Processing encounters, Move 4 of EFIT Tango
Move 5 of EFIT Tango. *See* Integration and validation, Move 5 of EFIT Tango
Mowrer, O. H., 18

N

Nervous system, structure in, 13
Nonpathologizing approach of EFT, 72–73, 104

O

Open-ended questions, 134, 181

P

Pacing, Accurate and on-target reflections, Collaborative process, Empathic attunement (PACE)
accurate and on-target reflections, 76–77, 105
collaborative process, 77–78, 105
empathic attunement and therapist presence, 77, 78, 105
pacing with attention to capacity, 76, 77, 105
Patterns, in EFT, 68
Paula case example, 9–11
PE. *See* Prolonged exposure
Perry, B. D., 2
Posttraumatic growth, 33
Posttraumatic Growth Inventory (PTGI), 33
Posttraumatic stress disorder (PTSD)
Barlow on, 8
dissociation, 28–29
due to sexual abuse before age 18, 7
as emotional disorder, 8
Janet's definition of, 4
secure attachment and supportive relationships for less symptoms of, 22
statistics, 3
Preparation for EFIT Tango, 37–38
Presence of therapist in EFT, 68
Present moment in EFT, 68
Primary/core affect in EFT, 68
A Primer for EFIT (Johnson and Campbell), 134
Process in EFT, 68
Processing encounters, Move 4 of EFIT Tango, 220
focus on key aspects of encounter, 46
Randy and Karen case example, 163

Saul case example, 126
Sierra case example, 91, 94, 99
summarization and validation, 46–47
validation and acknowledgement of fears, 47
Prolonged exposure (PE) therapy, 7
Protective factors, against impact of trauma experience, 4
Proxy voice, use of in EFT, 65, 69
Psychotherapy, 14
PTGI. *See* Posttraumatic Growth Inventory
PTSD. *See* Posttraumatic stress disorder
Purpose, sense of, meaning making, negative impact on, 6

Q

Questions
evocative, 38, 62, 65, 69
open-ended, 134, 181

R

Randy and Karen case example, 145–146, 149, 162–162, 170–171
Reactive anger, 78, 136
Reflecting present processes, Move 1 of EFIT Tango, 35, 105
asking evocative questions, 38
desired outcome, 39
focus on self of client, 38
focusing on connections with others, 38–39
process of emotion regulation, 39
Saul case example, 112
Sierra case example, 81, 86, 87, 88–89, 98
Reflection, micro intervention of EFT, 60–62, 64–65, 69
Reframing, micro intervention of EFT, 66, 69
Regulation capacity, affect, 229
Relational capacity, 147, 151, 157
Relational dramas, 2
Relational impacts, 135, 148, 157
Relational, shame is, 173
Relationship, in CARE, 76
Resilience, 4, 8, 45, 199, 204, 217
capacity for, 14, 53, 68, 139
increased from secure attachment, 23, 50, 72, 175
in secure connection, 30, 31, 52, 68
traumatic loss and, 209

Response
  broadening space between triggers and,
    95, 141, 142, 174, 187, 229, 231, 235
  therapist highlighting of triggers and,
    50, 116
  triggers and, 214, 219, 223
Restructuring, stage 2 in EFT, 59–60,
    68, 220
  anticipated outcomes, 229, 234–235
  connection to dissolve shame, 135–172
  deepened level of flexibility, 142
  grief emerges, 145
  identity epiphanies, 143
  Randy and Karen case example,
    145–171
  Sandy case example, 145
Rigidity, 187
  limited capacity and, 72
  shame shifts to flexibility from, 142,
    146, 153, 158–159, 165, 170
Rogers, Carl, 8, 53, 59
  on emotion organization of inner life
    and relationships, 18

S

Safe haven, principle of attachment, 22
  for each client in couple therapy, 27
  emotional connection, 21, 204
  single incident trauma and, 204
  therapeutic alliance, 70, 141, 151
Sandy case example, 144–145
Saul case example, 11, 106–107, 110,
    112–114, 116–117, 119, 121–124,
    126–133
Secondary strategies or styles, anxious
    dismissing attachment, 23
Second-level change, 5
Secrecy, 7
Secure attachment
  first responder trauma and, 198, 199
  grief emerging with client access to,
    145
  increased resilience from, 23, 50, 72,
    175
Secure base, principle of attachment, 22
Secure connection
  to heal trauma, goal of therapy, 53–54,
    68
  resilience in, 30, 31, 52, 68
  self-reinforcing aspect of, 20
  shaping of, 27
Security, sense of, 164
  mental health and, 23

Self, sense of, 85
  ARE with, 19
  disconnection with, 6, 7, 152
  imbued with shame, 137, 151–152,
    161, 172
  impact of trauma on, 3
Self-blame, 57, 74, 99
  first responder trauma, 203
  trauma survivors, 28, 31–32, 107, 138,
    171, 229
Self-reinforcing aspect of secure
    connection, 20
Self-sufficiency, human myth, 17
Shame
  access to self and experience with
    dissolution of, 142–143, 156,
    167–168
  adaptive in certain circumstances,
    136–137, 172
  AIRM and, 138–139, 172–173
  through attachment lens, 146–147, 172
  compassion as antidote to, 127, 142,
    162, 170, 173
  early cumulative experiences thwart
    development, 137–138, 149,
    152–153, 157, 172
  EFCT and EFIT differences and
    similarities, 173
  emotion links self and experience, 140,
    157, 173
  grief and sense of loss, 167–168, 173
  as inhibitor, 135, 155, 172
  key assumptions for EFT treatment of,
    173
  negative sense of self, 137, 151–152,
    161, 172
  prototypical responses shift from
    rigidity to flexibility, 142, 146, 153,
    158–159, 165, 170
  proximity to self offers starting point,
    140, 150, 173
  as relational, 135, 148, 157, 173
  stabilization stage 1, contextualization
    and restructuring stage 2, addressing
    of, 141–142, 173
  stillness facilitates immediacy,
    140–141, 157–158, 162, 173
  survivor guilt or moral injury, 137
  trauma survivors, 28
  ways out of, 172–173
Shame-based identity, 29
Shaver, Phillip, 17
Sierra case example, 81–100, 102–103,
    143–144

Single incident trauma
  safe haven relationship, 204
  special considerations in working with,
    218
  stalking victim assault, 206–207
  traffic accident, 204–205, 208–209
Soft, Slow, Simple, and Specific, in EFT,
    67
Softening, in EFT
  bonding events in EFCT, 17
  core vulnerabilities, 11
Stabilization, stage 1 in EFT, 59–60, 69,
    220
  anticipated outcomes, 224–225, 234
  finding focus and maintaining
    momentum, 106–134
  follow emotion or felt experience, 117,
    123, 134
  increased flexibility, 142
  lead client into and through emotion,
    111, 117–119, 134
  maintain focus, 110, 134
  Marjorie case example, 221–225
  prompt with open-ended questions, 134
  redirect as needed, 108, 113–114, 134
  resource client, 120, 134
  Sandy case example, 144
  summarize and reflect, 115, 119, 121,
    134
  tracking, validation and reflection,
    141–142, 221, 228
  transparency facilitates collaboration
    and choice, 134
  trust and access build, 143
  use of EFIT Tango as guide, 113, 134
  use self of therapist to maintain focus
    and momentum, 134
  validation, 127
  when client exits, validate and refocus,
    110, 117, 134
Stage 1 in EFT. See Stabilization, stage 1
  in EFT
Stage 2 in EFT. See Restructuring, stage
  2 in EFT
Stage 3 in EFT. See Consolidation, stage
  3 in EFT
Stalking victim assault as single incident
  trauma, 206–207
Stigma, 7
Suicidality, youth and electronic device
  use, 30
Supportive social networks as protective
  factor, 4
Survivor guilt, 137

T
Tavistock Clinic research, Bowlby and,
    16
Therapeutic alliance, 26, 67
  CARE relationship, 76
  safe haven principle, 70, 141, 151
Therapist
  acknowledges power of need for others,
    56–57, 68
  collaboration in ARE relationship, 54,
    68
  empathic attunement and presence in
    PACE, 77, 78, 105
  focus with CARE, 74–75, 104
  highlighting of triggers and response,
    50, 116
  presence in EFT, five Ps, 68
  stabilization stage 1, use of self to
    maintain focus, 108, 134
  tracking emotion in Move 2 of EFIT
    Tango, 39–40
Therapy
  empathic reflection, 2, 78, 105
Tracking
  emotion, Move 2 of EFIT Tango,
    39–40
  unfolding drama, Move 3 EFIT Tango,
    66–67
  validation and reflection, 141–142,
    221, 228
Traffic accident, as single incident
  trauma, 204–205, 208–209
Trauma
  closeness as dangerous, 125
  cumulative of first responder, 198,
    199–200
  defined, 2
  developmental, 3
  of emotional isolation, 16, 48
  emotions blocked by, 206
  existential focus of, 3
  felt experience of, 208
  freeze or flee response, 208
  lack of control as common with,
    159
  limited options for emotion regulation,
    23
  multidimensional nature of impacts
    of, 4
  perspective on, 2–5
  public awareness of, increase in, 3
  sense of self impacted, 3
  shame and self-disgust, 107

Trauma, assumptions for healing from
    client capability of growth and
        resilience if offered safety, 14, 53,
        68, 139
    corrective emotional experiences foster
        growth, 58–59, 68
    emotion is prioritized, 54–55, 68
    goal of secure connection with self and
        others, 53–54, 68
    therapist acknowledges power of need
        for others, 56–57, 68
    therapist collaboration with ARE, 54,
        68
    therapist resources client with self and
        others, 57, 68
    therapist tracks content and process,
        55–56, 68
Trauma recovery, core elements, 12
Trauma survivors
    labels and stigma, 28
    self-blame, 28, 31–32, 107, 138, 171,
        229
    shame and acceptance of blame, 28
Traumatic experiences
    despair, unmanageable emotional pain,
        6
    emotional isolation and loneliness, 6
    helplessness and lack of agency, 6–7
    through lens of attachment science, 13
    protective factors, 4
    self and world engagement change
        with, 2
Traumatic loss
    AIRM protocol, 216–217, 218
    change involvement with, 210–211, 218
    client grief and CARE, 213, 218
    as destabilizing, 209–210, 218
    grief as frequent visitor, 212, 218
    grief process, 211–212, 218
    guiding assumptions and
        considerations, 209–218
    identification of blocks to mobilize
        grief, 214–215
    resilience and, 209
    trauma addressed to make space for
        grief of, 215–216, 218
Traumatic memories, treatment exposure
    to, 7
Traumatic stress, treatment of
    Bertalanffy on levels of change, 5
    CBT, 7
    compelling negative emotions
        addressed, 7

    corrective emotional experience, 8
    CPT, 7
    dropout rates, 7
    EFCT and EFIT, 6
    EMDR, 7
    exposure to traumatic memories, 7
    PE, 7
Trauma trap, dysfunctional responses
    create, 2
Triggers, 149, 178, 234
    body sensation, 41, 87
    broadening space between response
        and, 95, 141, 142, 174, 187, 229,
        231, 235
    cognition/meaning, 41, 87
    elements of emotions, 40–41
    Move 2 of EFIT Tango, 41, 42, 87
    response and, 214, 219, 223
    therapist highlighting response to, 50,
        116
    therapist reflecting and repeating, 41,
        87

V

Validation
    of anger, 78–79
    of blocks, 44, 47, 51, 233
    in EFT stabilization stage 1, 110, 117,
        127, 134, 141–142, 221, 228
    micro intervention of EFT, 62–63, 69,
        141–142, 161
    Move 5 of EFIT Tango, integration
        and, 35, 47–48, 220

W

Waal, Frans de, 17
What Happened to You? (Perry and
    Winfrey), 2
Window of tolerance, capacity and, 51,
    75, 80, 89, 92, 94, 123, 199
Winfrey, O., 2
Work culture, first responder trauma
    protective factors from, 198
World Health Organization ICD-11, 6

Y

The Year of Magical Thinking (Didion),
    210–211
Yezda case example, 174–181, 194–195
Youth, electronic device use, 30